Coping with
DEMENTIA

A *handbook for carers*

 Health **E**ducation **B**oard for **S**cotland

About this HANDBOOK

This book contains information and advice for people who care for someone who has dementia. It aims to:
• help you feel less alone
• give you practical advice on coping
• help you to find caring more rewarding and less stressful
• show you where to go for help and for more information.

Every person with dementia is different. Dementia can bring many problems, but not all of them will happen to any one person. When you read through this book, remember that the person you care for will not experience everything you read about. This book is designed to help you cope, not to worry you!

If you want to talk about anything you have read, or would like more information or local contacts, you can call the 24 hour Dementia Helpline. The number is 0800 317 817 and all calls are free.

Note: As more women than men have dementia, we decided to call the person with dementia 'she' in this book. Using 'he or she' all the time can be awkward to read. However, the information applies just as much to men who have dementia.

ISBN 1 873452 81 0

© Health Education Board for Scotland 1996

Typeset in 11/14 Caslon 540

Designed by Mark Blackadder

Illustrations by Sheila Cant

616.83 (HEA)

CONTENTS

CONTENTS

CONTENTS

ACKNOWLEDGEMENTS

Section 1
ABOUT DEMENTIA

WHAT IS DEMENTIA?

Dementia is an illness of the brain. When someone has dementia, brain cells are damaged and die faster than they do normally. Losing brain cells means that the person's brain does not work as well as it should. Gradually she begins to lose the ability to do things. Often it affects memory first. The person may become confused about who people are, where she is and what day it is. Everyday tasks become more and more difficult. Her personality may change.

Dementia is progressive, and the person will get gradually less and less able. However, this usually happens slowly. The person will gradually need more help. Eventually someone with dementia will be unable to manage even basic tasks like eating, dressing and going to the toilet. But this will not happen suddenly. The illness can last many years.

At present there is no cure for dementia. But there is a lot you can do. This book is about how you can help.

Dementia affects about 2% of people aged 65 to 70, 9% of people aged 70–80 and about one person in five over 80. Because people are living longer now, there are more people with dementia. It can also affect people in their 40s or 50s or even younger, although this is rarer. This is called early onset dementia (or sometimes pre-senile dementia).

TYPES OF DEMENTIA

There are many diseases which can cause dementia. The best known is Alzheimer's disease. Alzheimer's disease probably causes more than half of all cases of dementia. When someone has Alzheimer's disease, individual brain cells are damaged. Over time more and more brain cells fail to work properly. The result is a slow decline of mental abilities.

Second most common are vascular dementias, including multi-infarct dementia. In these types of dementia, the blood supply to the brain is damaged in some way. In multi-infarct dementia, tiny 'strokes' (called infarcts) cut off the blood supply to small areas of the brain and the brain cells die. These strokes may be so small that no-one notices them at the time. But the person may get worse quite suddenly, and then not change until the next stroke. So the progression of the illness can happen in a step like way.

Other types of dementia include:

Alcohol-related dementia, including Korsakoff's syndrome. People with alcohol-related dementia should not drink alcohol, as this will make their dementia get worse. In some alcohol-related dementia, the progression of the illness will stop if the person stops drinking.

Lewy Body dementia. This dementia seems to be connected with Parkinson's disease. Some people with Parkinson's disease develop a form of dementia, but people with Lewy Body dementia don't necessarily get symptoms of Parkinson's. People with this kind of dementia may be more likely to have hallucinations or spells of distressed or disturbed behaviour. They can also be very sensitive to some drugs which are sometimes used to help behaviour problems.

Frontal lobe dementia and Pick's disease. This kind of dementia damages the part of the brain which helps you control what you are doing. The person may be more likely to do things at the wrong time or in the wrong place, which can be embarrassing for the carer. Memory loss is not as common in this kind of dementia.

Other kinds of dementia include AIDS related dementia and Creutzfeld-Jacob disease. Some people with Down's syndrome also develop dementia, often in middle age.

Different kinds of dementia can lead to different kinds of problem and each person with dementia is different. It is impossible to know exactly which problems the person you care for will face. This book looks at how to cope with many of the difficulties dementia can cause. But remember, not all of them will happen to the person you care for.

If you would like to know more about dementia, ask the person's doctor and see the Further information section on page 95.

WHAT CAUSES DEMENTIA?

Dementia is the result of physical illnesses which affect the brain. The different types of dementia have different causes. A great deal of medical research is looking at possible causes and cures.

Old age does not cause dementia. It is more common in very old people, but eighty per cent of people over 80 stay mentally alert. Most of us will become a little forgetful from time to time. This is quite normal.

Carers sometimes think that the illness started with a crisis such as the death of a partner or moving house. These events do not cause dementia, but they may make someone in the early stages more confused. She may find a new house very confusing, or her late partner may have been helping so much that no-one else noticed a problem.

As far as we know, too much or too little mental activity does not cause dementia.

WHAT IS NOT DEMENTIA—THE IMPORTANCE OF A PROPER DIAGNOSIS

If you know someone who is forgetful or confused, don't just assume it is dementia or 'just old age'. Try to persuade her to see a doctor. Memory loss and confusion are not always a sign of dementia. They can have a number of other causes. These include:
• Infections, such as chest or urinary tract infections.
• Medicines, such as sleeping pills. If the dose is wrong or if the person takes several medicines together, this can lead to symptoms just like those of dementia.
• General medical conditions such as heart or thyroid trouble.
• Hypothermia (when the body temperature drops to low).
• Depression.

These problems can all be successfully treated. The person's memory and mental function should then get back to normal.

A firm diagnosis can be hard to make in the early stages. But if the doctor finds no other reason for the symptoms, he or she may diagnose dementia. It can be hard to get the right help and advice until the person has a diagnosis.

The person's family doctor may refer her to a specialist for a diagnosis. Or the doctor may make a diagnosis. If you are not happy with the diagnosis, ask the doctor to refer the person to a specialist for a second opinion. (See pages 78–80) The booklet *Getting help from your doctor* gives useful information—see Further information.

THE PERSON WITH DEMENTIA

These days, many people are being diagnosed with dementia quite early on in the illness. This means that they are still able to understand what is happening. The person with dementia will probably need a lot of support, emotional as well as practical. Talk to the doctor or another health or social work professional about this. Perhaps the person could see a counsellor to help her cope.

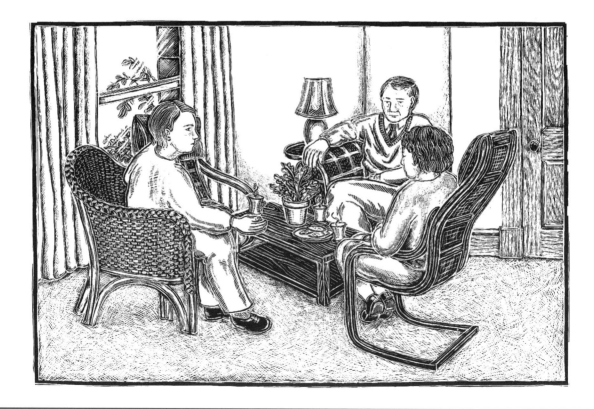

The person with dementia may be feeling depressed, frightened, frustrated or distressed. Try to give her reassurance. Later on in the illness the person will still have feelings even if it is hard to explain what she feels. It is important to recognise this. Although someone in the later stages of the illness may not remember an enjoyable event, she may still feel good afterwards.

If the person is still able to read, the booklet *Facing dementia* (see Further information) may be helpful. It is for people who have a diagnosis of dementia. It may help if someone reads it with the person, to help explain it.

Try to make sure that the person is as involved as possible in making decisions and choices about things that affect her. (See Money and legal matters, page 19.)

Don't be tempted to treat the person with dementia like a child. Even if she finds it hard to understand things, she is still an adult. She has a whole lifetime of experiences behind her, and an adult's needs, desires and rights.

HOW DEMENTIA PROGRESSES

The progress of the illness varies a lot from one person to another. This means that no-one can give firm answers about what you can expect. The problems can also vary from day to day or even hour to hour. Some changes are more common early in the illness and others tend to happen later, but this too is variable. The illness may last many years. It may sometimes progress faster in younger people.

At first, the changes are slight. The person with dementia may become forgetful and likely to repeat things. She may behave in ways which are a bit odd.

The person may be aware that something is wrong, and may be frightened that she is losing control. Some people become withdrawn and depressed, or agitated. The person may lose interest in life and find it hard to make day to day plans.

Only close family and friends may notice these changes.

One man with dementia described feeling as though a fog was covering his mind, making it hard to think clearly. Sometimes, on better days, the fog would lift, and some days it would get thicker.

As the illness goes on, the changes are greater. Behaviour which at first just seemed odd becomes hard to cope with. Memory problems get worse. The person may:
• confuse the time of day
• forget names of family or friends
• repeat questions over and over again
• not eat properly
• blame others for mistakes she has made
• neglect personal or home care
• wander about at night
• find it hard to grasp what is said
• need help with everyday tasks such as bathing and dressing
• be hard to understand at times, as she loses track of what she is saying or can't find the right words
• become angry or upset very quickly
• see or hear things that are not there (hallucinations).
These are all things which can go wrong when someone has dementia. But the person you care for probably won't have all these problems.

Many people become confused and lost, especially later in the illness. Often someone will not know even close family members. She may be quiet and withdrawn. The person will eventually need a great deal of help with eating, washing, bathing and using the toilet. She may become incontinent. Some people may be disturbed and restless at night.

The person's speech may make little sense. She may not understand what people say. But she may still understand some things. You may be able to communicate in other, non-verbal ways, such as through touch.

Some of the difficulties you may have faced earlier on will no longer be a problem. For example, if the person was frustrated and aggressive, she will probably be calmer. Some people with dementia seem quite calm later on in the illness. Someone may still be able to enjoy things at the time, even if she doesn't remember moments later; for example, a piece of familiar music, a smile or a hug.

By this time the person's personality may have changed a great deal. But she may keep well physically for a long time. Later, there is a marked physical decline which leads to death.

Having read this far you may be feeling very anxious about the future. Looking after a person with dementia can be hard, but there are many ways of making life easier and happier for both the person with dementia and yourself. This book draws on the experience of carers and we hope that the ideas will help you.

ABOUT DEMENTIA—SUMMARY

- Dementia is an illness of the brain.
- There are many diseases which can cause dementia.
- Each person with dementia is different.
- Not every problem will happen to the person you care for.
- Ask the doctor for more information.
- A proper diagnosis is very important.
- Remember the person with dementia's feelings and rights.

Section 2
COPING WITH CARING

Coping with CARING

EMOTIONAL REACTIONS

Looking after someone who has dementia can be very stressful. One of the things you may find hardest is living with your feelings about caring. It helps to know what these feelings might be.

Most carers experience a variety of emotions. The most common are sadness, guilt, anger and fear. Tiredness and tension are also common. Some of these feelings come as no surprise. You might expect to be sad when you feel you are slowly losing someone you love. Anger can be more of a shock. You may be alarmed at how frustrated and angry you can get. You may find you come to the end of your tether even over quite minor upsets.

On the other hand, caring can also be rewarding. For example, some people see it as a chance to give back to a parent the care they were given as a child. People with dementia often seem calm and happy despite the illness.

For many carers, there will be both rewarding and stressful times.

Many things can affect your reactions. For instance:
• Your relationship with the person with dementia. Someone you depended upon in the past may now be dependent on you. Or there may have been problems in your relationship in the past. Perhaps you are caring for your partner, and so no longer have the support you used to have in your relationship. You may miss things that kept you close, such as sharing problems and talking things out, or a sexual relationship.
• Your reasons for caring. People may find themselves looking after a relative because they want to, or from a sense of duty. Some may have little choice, which can add to the strain.
• Particular problems of the person you are caring for. For instance, night-time disturbance or constant demands for attention can be very stressful and tiring.
• Changes in your lifestyle. You may have given up a job, or moved to care for someone. You may be managing on less money than you used to have. You may feel isolated.

• How much support you have. Do you feel you are the only one looking after the person, or do other people share the care or share the responsibilities?

Caring for someone you don't live with brings its own worries too. Many people who care at a distance worry a lot about safety. Some people feel guilty about not being there all the time. Some feel frustrated because they find it hard to know what is going on.

It is useful to work out what makes you feel most upset. This will help you to be clear about the kind of help you need to keep up the care. Start by talking about the problems you are facing and your feelings. Look after yourself and share the job of caring.

What you can do

1. It helps if you talk about your feelings rather than bottle them up. You may want to do this with a friend or member of your family, or you may want to talk to a professional such as a social worker or community psychiatric nurse.

2. The 24 hour Dementia Helpline is always there on freephone 0800 317 817. Trained volunteers offer emotional support and information, whenever you want to call.

3. In most areas there are carers' support groups. Talking to others in the same situation can be a great help. Even if there is no support group nearby, it is still worth trying to meet with someone else who looks after someone with dementia. Other carers, more than anyone else, can understand what you are going through. Ask the Dementia Helpline or the social work department about groups in your area.

4. Some carers try to hide the fact that a relative has dementia. But dementia is an illness. It is not something to be ashamed of. It is not your fault, or your relative's. So try not to hide problems away or 'bottle them up'.

5. Don't assume that only the person you care for has a particular problem. Other carers have probably been through the same kind of thing.

6. Practise saying the right things to yourself. Research has shown that how you react to a problem—what you tell yourself—affects the way you feel. So learn the habit of telling yourself things that help you feel good. If the long term looks bleak take one day at a time.

Try not to give yourself negative messages like, 'If anything else happens I'll never manage,' or 'This is the last straw.' A more helpful approach is, 'I might not be doing a perfect job but I am doing quite well and getting better.'

You may find it more important to remind yourself of these things when you are feeling low. Changing the things you say to yourself can have an amazing effect on how you feel.

7. Don't be too hard on yourself. No-one is perfect. It is normal to lose your patience sometimes. If you lose your temper and shout at or hit the person, talk to someone right away. The Dementia Helpline can help you decide what to do to get help so that it doesn't happen again. Calls are confidential and you don't have to give your name.

When something goes wrong I say to myself, 'Relax, don't panic. I have coped so far and there is no reason why I won't continue to.' It seems to help, somehow.

At the beginning just after my wife was diagnosed I found things very hard. But I got through it. I used to tell myself, 'I can cope for today and that's all I need for today. Tomorrow can look after itself.'

EMOTIONAL REACTIONS: SUMMARY

- Caring can be both rewarding and stressful.
- Many things can affect your reactions.
- Talk about your feelings.
- The 24 hour Dementia Helpline is on freephone 0800 317 817.

• Join a carers' support group.
• Don't hide the fact that a relative has dementia.
• Don't assume that only the person you care for has a particular problem.
• Don't be too hard on yourself.

LOOK AFTER YOURSELF

1. Arrange for regular breaks to make sure you have time off. Friends, a local sitter service, day centres and day hospitals can help. (See page 72.)

2. Try not to become isolated from friends and family. This often happens if the person with dementia behaves in an embarrassing way or you can't leave her on her own. Explain the situation to friends and tell them that you do want them to visit. Most will be glad to help and will soon get used to any unusual behaviour.

3. Ask for respite breaks, to give you a weekend, a week or more away from taking care of the person with dementia. This gives you the chance to recharge your batteries.

4. Take time for yourself. Think about what you find relaxing. For example, it might be listening to music, watching television, going for a walk, seeing friends or something else. Try to make sure you get some time each day to relax, even if it's only a few minutes.

5. Looking after yourself is not selfish—it's sensible. You need to look after yourself, physically and emotionally, if you want to be able to go on caring.

My mother used to follow me absolutely everywhere and I never had a moment to myself. I took to locking myself in the bathroom for half an hour when things got too much. I took a book with me and put my headphones on and just left him to it.

LOOK AFTER YOURSELF—SUMMARY

• Give yourself a break.
• Explain the situation to friends and family.
• Take time for yourself every day.

• Remember, looking after yourself is not selfish—it's sensible.

YOU AND YOUR FAMILY

For many carers, looking after someone with dementia brings changes in family relationships. Perhaps you have children who are also having to cope with the person's illness. But the time you spend caring can mean less time looking after them. Perhaps your children feel embarrassed to bring their friends to the house. They may worry about what the person might do. Perhaps you feel you are doing more than some other family members and resent that. Or maybe the rest of the family worry about you wearing yourself out.

There may be no simple solution. But there are some ideas which may help.

What you can do

1. Many people with dementia enjoy spending time with children and the children enjoy it too. Talk to children or grandchildren about the illness. Try to explain that any odd behaviour is not the person's fault. It is because she is ill. Offer to explain this to their friends too.

2. Try to arrange some times when the person with dementia is out of the house so that children can see their friends. Perhaps she could go out with a friend or a home support worker sometimes.

3. Try not to let caring take over family life completely. Ask for help to give you time off to spend with your family. (See Getting help.)

4. Talk to the rest of the family. Relatives not involved in day-to-day caring may not realise the demands on you. They may not understand the illness. Perhaps you could have a family discussion about how to care for the person with dementia.

5. If there are disagreements on what is best, it may help to ask someone else to take part in discussions, to make sure

everyone gets a fair hearing. Perhaps a close friend, social worker, minister or the doctor could help.

My husband is sometimes very good with our grand-children, but sometimes he gets angry and they don't see why. The older ones understand a bit, but the youngest is only three and gets upset. I don't leave him alone with her any more. But I make sure they get times together doing something they enjoy and then I take her away again before he gets frustrated.

YOU AND YOUR FAMILY—SUMMARY

1. Talk to the whole family about the illness.
2. Try to arrange some times when children can see their friends.
3. Try not to let caring take over family life completely.

GETTING INFORMATION

It is easier to deal with caring when you have enough information. You may need information on the illness itself

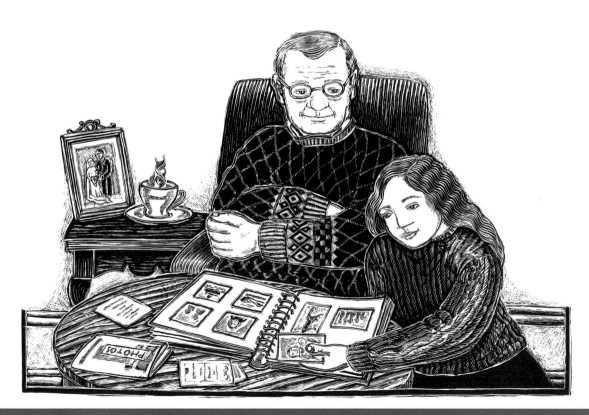

and how it will affect the person. You may need to find out about local services. Or you may want extra help with a particular problem.

I was at a meeting with various professionals talking about my wife's dementia and they all seemed to talk in initials! 'CPN' this and 'OT' that. Finally I just told them that if they wanted to get any sense out of me they'd have to speak English. They all looked very embarrassed and apologised for using jargon.

Dementia Helpline

The 24 hour Dementia Helpline on freephone 0800 317 817 can provide information on almost anything. If the person who takes your call can't answer a question, he or she will try to find out. The Dementia Helpline is run by Alzheimer Scotland—Action on Dementia and has a panel of expert advisers.

Carers' education

Although caring can be a full time job, few carers get any training in how to do it. So you may feel you have to learn by trial and error. Alzheimer Scotland—Action on Dementia and some other organisations organise carers' education through their local services. A carers' education course can give you the chance to get accurate information about the illness and how to cope. Research has shown that carers with this sort of training may feel less stressed than other carers. Call the Dementia Helpline to find out about a contact near you.

SHARE THE CARE

Looking after someone with dementia can be a round-the-clock job. No-one can provide all of the care, all of the time. Don't feel bad about accepting help. The help you need will change as time goes on. Get help as early on as possible. You may not feel you need much help now. But the person may find it easier to get to know a home support worker, for example, earlier on in the illness.

1. If possible, involve the person with dementia in discussions about her care. Try to make sure her wishes are heard.

2. If you can, try to share caring with other members of the family and friends.

3. Often people don't get help because no-one realises they need it. So it is important to ask. Friends and neighbours may be more willing to help than you expect once you explain things to them.

4.Regular help with shopping, housework and caring for the person with dementia will allow you time for yourself. The person with dementia will gain from having different company too.

5. Ask the social work department and doctor about what services are available. Ask the social work department for a community care assessment. (See Getting help, page 72) It is important for both you and the person with dementia that you make full use of these services.

6. There may come a time when it is no longer possible to care for the person with dementia at home. She may need residential, nursing home or hospital care. It can be hard to decide when this time has come. You may find it easier to decide if you discuss it with other members of the family or professionals. If the person goes into a hospital or home, you can still help care for her if you want to. (See Long-stay care, page 89.)

SHARE THE CARE - SUMMARY

• Try to share caring with other members of the family and friends.
• Involve the person in discussions about her care.
• Ask the social work department and doctor about what services are available.
• If you can no longer care for the person at home, discuss options with other members of the family and professionals.

Section 3
MONEY AND LEGAL MATTERS

PLANNING FOR THE FUTURE

When you find out that someone you are close to has dementia, it can be very upsetting. Often practical arrangements for the future are the last thing you and the person may think about. But it is a good idea to try to make plans sooner rather than later. That way the person with dementia can be as involved as possible in making choices. It is easier to deal with money and legal matters at the start of the illness, while the person is mentally capable of making decisions. It can be much harder to make arrangements later.

If the person can, she should make some important decisions as soon as possible. She should:
• write a will
• choose one or two people to look after her financial affairs if she becomes unable to, and give them a power of attorney
• make sure you and the doctor know of any wishes about medical care in the future—she could write this down as an advance directive or 'living will'.

Caring for a person with dementia at home can be quite costly. Financial benefits may be available. Some are available whatever the person's income or savings.

As time goes on, the person will become less able to cope with money. She may forget to pay bills, pay them twice, give money away or lose it. In time you may have to take on more of these tasks.

More information about these and other practical issues is in the booklets *Dementia: Money and Legal Matters* and *Facing Dementia* (see Further information).

WHAT YOU CAN DO

1. If the person has no bank account, encourage her to open one. Talk to the bank manager, who may arrange a mandate for the person with dementia to sign. This would let you use the account on her behalf.

2. Arrange direct debits so that the bank pays all bills

automatically. Gas, electricity and telephone companies and other organisations can help with this.

3. If the person is severely mentally impaired, she may get a discount on the council tax. Some carers can get a discount too. People on a low income may get a council tax rebate. Ask the local council for details.

4. Encourage the person to make a will through her lawyer as soon as possible, so that she can choose what happens to her money and possessions. A will is only valid if made when the person is clearly aware of what she is doing, so it is important not to put it off too long.

5. Encourage the person to give a power of attorney to someone she trusts. This may be you or someone else. It will give the power to handle the person's financial affairs. The person can only grant a power of attorney while she is still mentally capable. It may be a good idea to give two people a joint power of attorney. The document must be drawn up by a lawyer. Powers of attorney signed after 1st January 1991 remain valid as the person's illness progresses.

6. If the person with dementia loses money, gives it away, or forgets that she has spent it, he or she may accuse others of taking it. This can be distressing, but it is because of the illness. Reassure the person that he or she has enough money. Make sure the person always has some cash, even if it is a small amount. This may reassure her and help her keep some independence.

7. You can collect the person's pension and other benefits if she authorises you. If she can't sign or doesn't understand what she is signing, ask the Benefits Agency to make you (or someone else) her appointee. As appointee, you can apply for and collect all benefits on behalf of the person. You must tell the Benefits Agency if the person's situation changes.

8. The Benefits Agency can pay the retirement pension and most benefits directly into a bank account. This can be useful if you have arranged for the bank to pay the bills.

9. If the person is too confused she will not be able to grant a power of attorney. If there is no power of attorney there may be a problem. No-one will have the power to take money out of her account or to sell her house, for example. In some cases, the person may need a curator bonis appointed by the court to look after her money. This is an expensive and complicated procedure. If you think it is necessary, call the Dementia Helpline for information or ask a lawyer.

10. If you handle the person's money, always keep it separate from your own. Keep a record of what you receive and spend, in case someone asks you to account for it.

11. There are many other legal issues which might concern carers, such as giving consent for treatment. If you want advice contact your local Citizen Advice Bureau or see a lawyer. Lawyers will charge for any arrangement they make, but most will give advice free. Ask what their services will cost. You or the person with dementia may be entitled to Legal Aid.

BENEFITS

The person with dementia is probably entitled to benefits from the Benefits Agency. If she needs care or supervision, she may qualify for attendance allowance (if she is over 65) or disability living allowance (if he or she is under 65). These two benefits do not depend on the person's income. You and the person with dementia may be able to get other benefits too. For example invalid care allowance helps carers below retirement age, and income support helps people with a low income. Call the Benefits Enquiry Line for People with Disabilities free on 0800 882 200 for information. Or you can ask the welfare rights officer at the social work department or a Citizen's Advice Bureau. Don't hesitate to claim—remember, caring for someone with dementia is expensive. You have a right to benefits.

If the person is under 66

If the person is under 66, apply as soon as possible for disability living allowance. This is because it can help with *both* care needs and mobility needs. It is normally paid for the first time only if someone is under 65, but the claim can be backdated in some cases. Attendance allowance, for people over 65, does not help with mobility needs. If the person gets disability living allowance, she will still get it even when she passes 65.

Someone who gets disability living allowance to help with mobility needs may be exempt from road tax if a car is registered in her name, even if someone else does the driving.

Filling in forms

The forms for attendance allowance and disability allowance are very long. They ask for a lot of detail about the help the person needs. Get help filling in the form if you can. Ask your local Alzheimer Scotland—Action on Dementia project or Citizens Advice Bureau for help. Or use the Benefits Enquiry line. They can fill it in for you over the telephone. Give as much detail as you can. For example, if the person is not safe alone, give examples of what has happened or might happen.

If the person does not get the allowance you should consider making an appeal. Many people get it if they appeal. Don't make a new claim because it won't be backdated.

MONEY & LEGAL MATTERS: SUMMARY

- Encourage the person to open a bank account.
- Arrange to pay bills automatically.
- Encourage the person to grant a power of attorney if she can.
- Encourage the person to write a will if she can.
- Ask about welfare benefits and council tax discounts.
- Make sure the person has some cash.
- Keep the person's money separate from your own.

Money and Legal MATTERS

Section 4
PRACTICAL CARING

Every person with dementia is different, and will be affected differently by the illness. This section looks at some of the challenges and problems you and the person with dementia may face.

Remember, not every problem will happen to any one person. Remember too that things will change as the illness progresses. A difficulty which seems impossible to solve may just disappear with time.

For a while my mother kept losing her purse. She would get very upset and accuse me or her home help of stealing it. But she has become much calmer over the last few months. She doesn't look for her purse at all any more.

It helps if you have a good idea of what to do when a problem arises. There is a great deal that you can do to make things better for yourself and the person with dementia.

The What you can do sections list some practical ways of dealing with the changes which people with dementia go through. Finding the best way of coping is often a matter of trial and error. But these ideas have helped other carers.

Don't feel you have to cope on your own. Call the 24 hour Dementia Helpline for suggestions of how to approach a problem. Or talk to the person's doctor, community psychiatric nurse, occupational therapist and to other carers.

LOOKING AFTER THE PERSON

Each person with dementia is an individual and has her own lifestyle and experiences. Try to remember this when you are caring. Try to help the person to carry on with existing interests and social activities as much as possible.

Activities

Each person with dementia will enjoy different activities, according to her interests and how the illness is affecting her. You may have to help more with an activity, or simplify it as time goes on. Try to find things for the person to do which she can succeed with. A feeling of failure can be very distressing.

Don't feel you must provide something to do every minute of the day. Quiet time is important too. Sometimes the job of caring for someone with dementia takes up so much time and energy that it's hard to fit in enjoyable activities. Try to find help with caring so that you are under less pressure. A day centre can offer enjoyable and stimulating activities for the person and give you time off. See Getting help.

Talk to other carers and see books on activities for ideas (see Further information).

What you can do

1. Think about what the person used to enjoy for ideas on what to try. Try to help the person you care for to keep doing things she used to do.

2. Many people with dementia can still remember things that happened a long time ago, even if they can't remember more recent events. So they may enjoy activities like looking through old family photographs or copies of old newspapers, for example.

3. Help the person to make a 'life story book'. This could be a scrapbook with reminders of important times in her life, such as photographs, tickets, postcards and so on. The book can be enjoyable to make, and it can help

professional workers get to know the person better too. The person may enjoy just looking through the book later.

4. Many people with dementia like to feel useful, and may enjoy helping around the house.

5. Many people will enjoy listening to familiar music.

6. Remember that even if the person doesn't remember an activity, it is still worthwhile if she enjoys it at the time.

My mother loves to dust. She sometimes does the mantelpiece over and over again, but she gets a lot of satisfaction out of it, so I don't stop her.

My father used to go down to the bowling club every week. He stopped going for a while because he was worried that his pals wouldn't accept him because he has Alzheimer's disease. When he told me I asked if he minded me talking to them. He said that was OK, and now a couple of them come round every week and drive him there.

Until she had her first stroke, my sister used to be an avid bridge player. She still loves to play cards, so now we play snap and other simple games.

Spiritual well-being

Caring for the whole person with dementia means caring for spiritual needs too. Most people's spirituality is to do with their ethnic culture, tradition and upbringing.

A person's individual awareness of her place and purpose in creation is unique. This is the person's spirituality. People have different personal ways of finding a sense of spiritual well-being. If spirituality has been important to someone, it is important to help her to have contact with things that in the past were part of her spiritual well-being. Without this, some people may feel abandoned. They may feel a sense of loss of worth and purpose.

What you can do

1. Find out what spiritual things if any used to be important to the person. For example, this may include religious worship, meditation, books, songs or chants, symbols, places or other things.

2. If the person attended religious worship or groups or festivals, try to help her to keep attending for as long as possible. If this becomes impossible, perhaps she can continue to take part in worship at home.

3. Help the person to stay in contact with other people from her place of worship. Encourage visitors.

4. Help the person to feel that she still belongs, for example by reading newsletters or magazines from the church, mosque, synagogue, temple or other place of worship.

5. Help the person with personal devotion. For example, familiar readings from holy books, prayers or meditation.

6. Ask the person's minister, priest, rabbi, imam or other religious leader or teacher to visit to give pastoral care to the person, and to you if you wish.

Although my aunt doesn't speak any more, she still loves to sing hymns and remembers every word.

LOOKING AFTER THE PERSON—SUMMARY

Activities

- Try to help the person keep doing things she used to do.
- Try activities that let the person use older memories.
- Help the person to make a 'life story book'.
- The person may enjoy helping around the house.
- Find out about day centres.

Spiritual well-being

- Find out what used to be important to the person.
- Try to help her to keep attending religious worship.
- Help the person to stay in contact with other people and

newsletters from her place of worship.
- Help the person with personal devotion.
- Ask for pastoral care.

LOSS OF MENTAL ABILITIES

Forgetfulness

Most people with dementia will have memory problems. Usually these are mild at first, and simple memory aids may be very helpful. Later on in the illness the person with dementia may become more confused and 'lost' or disorientated. She may forget basic facts such as who other people are, where they are and what year it is. She may confuse the past with the present.

My sister gets anxious sometimes and wants to go home to look after her children. She's forgotten that they're grown up with children of their own now.

Early on in the illness there are simple practical ways to jog the person's memory. The following ideas will help you and the person with dementia cope with forgetfulness. They will help the person keep her mind alert for as long as possible. This approach is known as reality orientation. It means providing reminders to help the person keep an idea of where she is, who people are, what time of day it is, what season it is and so on.

Reassurance is very important. The person may be aware that she now can't remember what she used to. This can be upsetting, frightening and frustrating. Try to be reassuring. Respond to the emotions the person shows as well as to what she actually says or does.

Later in the illness memory aids probably won't help. You will need to give more direct reminders and help.

What you can do

1. Keep to routines as much as you can and try not to change where things are. Being in familiar surroundings helps. Changes can make confusion worse.

2. A useful routine may be to plan the day's events at breakfast time. Try getting the person with dementia to write these down in a diary. Then go over the diary again at lunch time.

3. Get a large clock with the day and date. A loud tick helps remind the person with dementia where the clock is. Put up a calendar and mark off the days.

4. Put signs in words or pictures on doors to help the person find the way around. Or just leave doors open so that the person can see what's in each room.

5. Use a memory board or notice board as a reminder of what is going on. Put it somewhere it is easy to see, such as in the kitchen.

6. You will need to draw the person's attention to memory aids and check that she understands them. The aids alone don't work. Remind her to look at the memory board, calendar, diary and signs. Leave notes where the person will see them.

7. If you are not with the person, you can make sure that she remembers things by phoning.

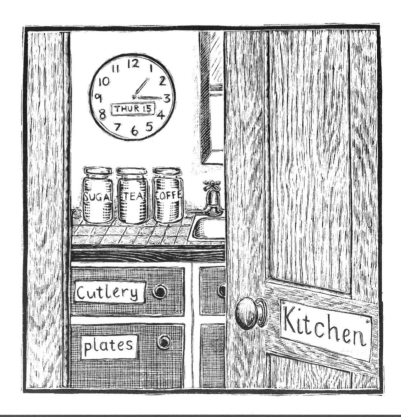

8. You may need to provide basic facts in your conversation such as reminders about time, place and people. Helpful facts might include who you are, where she is, where you are going, what is happening and so on. Be tactful and don't wait for the person to fail.

9. Family photographs, including photographs of the person with dementia, can help her keep a sense of identity. Talk about them, particularly if her sight is not good. Named photos of regular visitors (family, friends, home help) may help her to know people when they call.

10. Memory aids work best when the person is in the habit of using them; for example, if she has always used a diary. Tryto help her get into the habit as early as you can in the illness. Get other people who visit to write in the diary too.

11. Ask the social work department or hospital to refer the person with dementia to an occupational therapist for practical advice (see page 84).

Whenever I go out I leave a note for my wife on the door of the fridge to say when I'll be back. Before I go I point it out to her and get her to read it to me by asking if she can read my writing, just to make sure she understands.

To help my brother keep track of time, I'll usually drop something into the conversation like, 'Oh good—it's Saturday—but isn't it cold for October!'.

Sometimes my Dad would mention a visitor he'd had, but he was never sure who it was. So I put out a 'visitor's book' and asked people to sign in. It turned out that the mystery person was his care worker.

Repeated questioning

Some people with dementia keep asking the same question over and over again. This is because the person simply does not remember asking. Many carers find this very difficult to deal with. It can be frustrating and irritating, especially if the person follows you around the house asking questions. The person may seem afraid to let you out of sight. She may not be able to remember where you are or whether you will be back.

What you can do

1. Remind yourself that the person really does forget having asked a question before, or forgets the answer. Remember that she is not doing it deliberately to annoy you.

2. Be tactful. For example it is better to say, 'Oh, didn't I mention that we're going to the shops to buy bread and milk,' rather than 'I've told you that already.'

3. Be reassuring, The person may be asking because she is anxious about something. Try reassuring her physically, perhaps with a hug.

4. Try writing the answer to the question in a notebook or on a noticeboard. Point it out as you answer. Try to help the person get used to looking there for the answer.

5. Keep the person involved in what is happening. Make eye contact when you talk to her. Remember to include the person with dementia if there is a group conversation. This will help lessen anxiety and may reduce questions.

6. Use the memory aids suggested. (See page 31)

7. Try to divert her attention and involve her in another activity.

8. Even with all your efforts she may keep repeating questions. You may have to leave the room to keep your patience.

He used to ask the same thing again and again and it used to drive me round the bend sometimes. It was usually about when the bus for the day centre was coming, what time was dinner, things like that. So now I try to remind him about things as I talk, and I put up reminders on the fridge door. He still asks, but not as often. I can either answer or just point to the fridge. It helps me keep my patience longer.

Conversation and communication

As dementia gets worse communication becomes a problem. You may find that the person seems deaf at times. Deafness may be the problem, but it is also likely that the person hears but does not understand. Dementia slows people down in their ability to take things in and make sense of what they hear. Some people may have difficulty finding the right words for what they want to say. They may also begin to lose track of what they are saying in the middle of a sentence. It becomes harder to hold a conversation. This can be very frustrating for both people with dementia and carers.

What you can do

1. Make sure that the person's dentures, glasses or hearing aid are in good working order and are the correct prescription. Poor sight and hearing can make people more confused and conversation difficult.

2. Speak clearly, simply and slowly but don't shout. Make sure the person can see your face when you speak.

3. Try to get one idea across at a time.

4. You may have to repeat yourself. Sometimes it helps if you say things slightly differently the second time:
'Your sister Freda is coming to tea today.'
'We're having a visitor this afternoon. Your sister Freda is coming.'

5. Use closed questions which ask for a simple answer. *Instead of asking my grandmother, 'What would you like to do this afternoon?', I'll say, 'Do you want to go for a walk, or shall we look at some photographs?'.*

6. Allow plenty of time for the person to take in what you say and to reply.

7. Try not to confuse or embarrass the person by correcting her bluntly.

8. If the person with dementia cannot find the right words, ask her to describe what she means and suggest a word.

But don't get into the habit of providing the right word as soon as she hesitates. If you do, she may become less confident. She might give up trying. Be encouraging but let her know you understand how frustrating it is trying to find the right words.

9. Guess what the person is trying to say. Always ask if your guess is right. This is especially important when you are trying to understand what the person feels. She may not be able to say why she feels worried, sad, angry or unhappy. If you do manage to grasp the feeling, let her know this. It will help to lessen feelings of being alone and isolated.

It was hard to know what was upsetting my husband. He wasn't able to say. Then at bed-time I noticed his toe was badly swollen.

10. A smile, touch or gesture can be just as important in getting the message across and showing that you care. Holding the person's hand when you talk can also be very reassuring.

11. Many people with dementia enjoy talking about the past. You may both enjoy reliving some of these memories together. Talking about things which she remembers well may help the person to feel secure. Try to make sure that she doesn't confuse these memories with the present. You can do this by making comparisons with how things were then and now.

Confused thinking

As dementia progresses the person's thinking becomes more mixed up. She may confuse memories of the past with the present. She may confuse facts with imaginings. As well as using memory aids, there are some good ways of trying to deal with confused thinking.

Dementia can cause difficulties with abstract thought as well as memory problems. For example, the person may find it harder to understand emotions or humour. She may take things literally.

Don't agree with confused thinking. This can just make it worse. But you don't always have to try to put the person right. Use a flexible approach, depending on the situation.

What you can try

1. Try disagreeing tactfully to correct the confusion. No-one likes to be corrected too often, so you have to be careful with this approach. Sometimes it can lead to upset. You will have to play it by ear.

2. Don't confront the person. Try diverting her onto another subject until she forgets.

3. Respond kindly to the person's feelings without agreeing with what she is saying.

'Another beautiful day,' my mother would say on coming down for breakfast—often with the rain lashing down! And I would simply say, 'You're feeling good then?'

My partner sometimes gets mixed up about what year it is. Sometimes he goes back in his mind to when he was working and gets anxious about getting to work on time. The first few times I told him that he doesn't work any more but he'd insist he does and we'd end up arguing. So now I reassure him that it's all right, he doesn't have to go to work today.

LOSS OF MENTAL ABILITIES—SUMMARY

Forgetfulness

- Keep to routines and don't make changes unless you have to.
- Use memory aids and draw attention to them.
- Drop reminders into your conversation.
- Go over a diary each day.
- Use familiar objects to help reassure the person about her past.
- Ask an occupational therapist for practical advice.

Repeated questions

- Remember that repeated questions are not meant to annoy you; they need repeated answers.

- Try to be patient, tactful and reassuring.
- Try other ways of reminding the person of the answer, such as a notebook.
- Try to change the subject gently.
- Keep the person with dementia involved in what is happening.

Conversation and communication

- Check dentures, hearing aids and glasses.
- Face the person, speak clearly and use simple sentences.
- Be patient and allow extra time.
- Help with word-finding problems.
- Use touch and gesture.
- Let the person know that you understand how frustrating it is.
- You may have to repeat yourself slightly differently.
- Use closed questions.
- Try not to embarrass the person.

Confused thinking

- Try not to go along with confused thinking, but be flexible.
- Sometimes gentle correction works.
- Use distraction.
- Talk about feelings the person is showing.

DAILY LIVING

People with dementia usually find everyday tasks such as dressing or eating gradually harder as time goes on. So they need more help. If you can, try to help the person with dementia to do things rather than doing them yourself. This can take more time, but it helps the person keep as independent as possible. You may have to find a balance between time and effort for you and independence for the person.

Dressing

People with dementia often have problems with dressing. They may lose track of the order of putting on clothes or forget half-way through and start to undress. They may struggle with fastenings and give up easily. The person may need help but not want it. For all these reasons dressing can take a long time.

What you can do

1. Allow plenty of time for the person to get dressed. If rushed she may become more confused and upset. Make sure the room is warm and she has used the toilet first.

2. As a general rule avoid doing too much for the person. Encourage her to do things for herself. This will help keep up self-esteem and confidence. Remind her what to do next if necessary. If that doesn't work, try showing her with actions. Break actions down into small steps.

3. Allow the person some choice, even if it is limited.

4. Lay out clothes in the order she will put them on. If possible, keep to the order that the person was in the habit of using.

5. If the person tries to put something on the wrong way, tactfully correct her and give help. Explain what you are doing. The more patient you can be the less likely the person is to become irritable and uncooperative.

6. If you have to do most of the dressing for the person, start by putting clothes on either the top or bottom half of

her body, then the other half. Don't at any time leave her entirely naked.

7. If the person has had a stroke, this may have left a weakness in a limb. It is much easier to place the weak limb into an item of clothing first and take it out last.

8. Buttons and hooks may be difficult. You can often replace them with zips or Velcro. Bras are easier to manage if they fasten at the front. Consider self-support stockings or socks.

9. If the person is incontinent and quite dependent for help with dressing, some carers find that track suit tops and trousers can be very useful. They are practical, easy to change, quick to wash and dry and they don't need ironing. For information about special designs of clothing, contact Disability Scotland. (See page 96.)

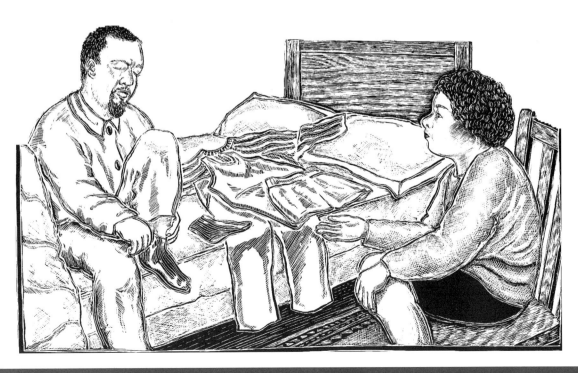

10. The person should only wear slippers for short times. Well-fitting shoes give support and reduce the risk of foot problems.

11. Put clothes for washing out of sight so that the person does not put them on again.

When my Dad saw all his shirts in the cupboard he just couldn't choose and got confused and upset. So I put most of them in a different place and just left him a couple of his favourites. Now he picks the shirt he's going to wear quite happily.

Every time I visited my mother she was wearing exactly the same clothes. She had plenty of other things in her wardrobe but she wouldn't wear them. We'd argue when I tried to get her to change. So I bought some more clothes the same as the ones she likes. She doesn't notice when I put out the clean ones while she's in bed. Now she's cleaner and we're both more relaxed because I've stopped nagging her.

I used to spend so long prompting my mother to dress herself that it became the main activity of the morning. Now we compromise. I help her a bit more, and with the time saved we go out for a walk or do something else we both enjoy.

Appearance and personal care

In time dementia causes the person to forget how to do even basic tasks of personal care. She may forget to clean her teeth or comb her hair, cutting nails may be a problem. For men shaving may be a problem. The person may lose interest in how she looks. Of course, many people with dementia do not like to be reminded about these personal tasks. But it is important to encourage the person to do as much as possible for herself.

What you can do

1. Take notice and compliment the person when she looks good. When she needs help or prompting, be tactful. Criticism or nagging may upset the person.

2. Remind the person when necessary about cleaning teeth. It may help if you clean your teeth at the same time

to remind her what to do. You may need to clean the person's teeth or dentures as her memory gets worse.

3. Dental care is vital. Ensure regular check-ups. Ask about the home dental service if visits to the dentist become too difficult. (Contact your health board if the person's own dentist is unable to visit.)

4. Remember to check finger and toe nails regularly. Cut them if the person can't. If you can't cut them arrange for a chiropody visit. (See page 85.)

5. A trip to the hairdressers, or a shampoo and set at home may help the person feel good. So can make-up and nail varnish.

6. Men may need to be reminded to shave each morning. Using an electric shaver is safer and may allow the person to shave himself independently for longer. Later in the illness he may find it hard to learn to use a new kind of razor. If he keeps using a traditional razor, you will soon have to supervise shaving. You may even have to do it for him.

My brother will rarely open his mouth to let me brush his back teeth. But he usually lets me brush the front ones. My mother gets a great boost from her fortnightly trip to the hairdresser. I also try to make sure she has a touch of makeup and nail varnish. She always used to wear it and I think it makes her feel more self-confident.

Bathing

It may be difficult to persuade the person with dementia to have a bath. She may protest that she has just taken one. Bathing itself can have its problems. Some people forget how to wash themselves, wash one area several times and forget others, forget to use soap, or forget to rinse off the soap. The person may not like being supervised.

What you can do

1. Try to make bath time as pleasant as possible. Allow plenty of time and ensure that the bathroom is warm. All

sorts of little things might help to make bathing more relaxed. Try music or bubble bath, for example.

2. Use a non-slip rubber mat in the bath and ensure that the flooring beside the bath is non-slip.

3. You may have to help the person in and out of the bath. Various aids may be available. A bath seat might help. Hand rails on the side of the bath make it easier for the person to get in and out. Ask the occupational therapist or nurse. (See page 84.)

4. People with dementia may have problems with the lock on the bathroom door. If this happens you could remove the lock. Replace it with one that can be unlocked from both sides or move it to a part of the door where the person is unlikely to use it.

5. Later in the illness you will need to supervise bathing all the time. Reassure the person that you are there to help. Put a chair beside the bath for yourself.

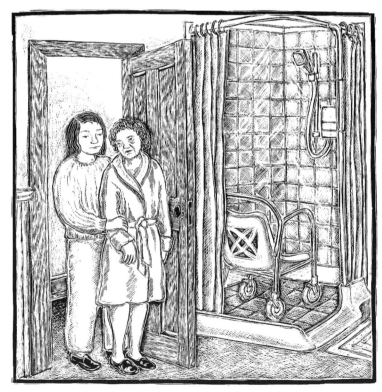

6. There are many new shower unit designs which some carers find useful. Ask the occupational therapist. But the person with dementia may be upset by a shower if she is not used to them.

7. Think about whether the person has to have a bath. Is it necessary for hygiene, or would an all-over wash do instead?

8. If you cannot deal with bathing or showering, for example if you need to lift the person, ask your health visitor, doctor or social worker for advice. Sometimes the district nurse or a home care assistant may be able to call in and help. Different areas have different arrangements for bathing services. People who go to a day hospital can be bathed there if bathing at home is impossible.

My Dad was very unwilling to have a bath. I think he was embarrassed for his daughter to see him naked. I talked to the day hospital he goes to and they agreed to try. The nurse had no problem at all persuading him to bath with her help!

Managing continence

Some people with dementia may become incontinent of urine (wet themselves). Bowel incontinence is not common until very late in the illness.

If the person becomes incontinent, don't just accept it as part of the illness. Often the person may not be truly incontinent at all. She may have forgotten the way to the toilet or how to recognise the toilet. Or she may not recognise the feeling of a full bladder. Helping the person may solve the problem.

Incontinence of urine may be the result of an infection or some physical problem. For instance, in men it may be caused by an enlarged prostate gland. Infections can be treated. Physical problems can often be put right. Consult the person's doctor or community nurse.

Sadly, sometimes incontinence is because of the degree of brain failure in dementia. In this case, it cannot be cured and slowly gets worse. In the end the person may need changes of clothes through the day and bed-linen at night. Ask the doctor if there is a continence adviser in your area and ask about incontinence aids.

What you can do

1. Consult the doctor about the problem. Ask for an explanation of the cause, after she has examined the person and done tests.

2. If the incontinence cannot be treated, ask for an assessment by the community nurse. He or she can supply appropriate aids such as pads, pants and protective bedding. Don't just go out and buy your own supplies. The person is entitled to incontinence equipment if she has a medical need.

3. Watch for any restlessness or agitation. These may be signs that the person needs to go to the toilet, but she may not realise this.

4. To reduce embarrassment, take a very matter-of-fact approach. Avoid making an issue out of the problem.

5. It may help if you remind the person to go to the toilet at regular intervals. The timing will vary from person to person. Try keeping a chart of when she needs the toilet to help work out a routine.

6. It may help to have a sign on the toilet door, or just to leave the door open. Leave a light on at night to help the person find the way.

7. Zips or buttons may be too awkward for the person to manage. If this is a problem, clothes with Velcro fastenings might help.

8. If the toilet is not easy to reach, it may help to have a commode. Ask the community nurse.

9. It is dangerous for anyone who is incontinent to use a standard electric blanket. Special blankets are available, although they cost more.

10. Sometimes soiling is caused by severe constipation. Constipation may be caused by a poor diet. A well-balanced diet with plenty of fibre (roughage), such as fruit, vegetables, wholewheat bread and cereals helps prevent constipation. Make sure the person has enough to drink. This also helps prevent constipation. Don't use laxatives unless the doctor has prescribed them.

11. In some areas there is a laundry service to help with soiled linen. Contact your local social work office.

My mother sometimes came back from the day centre having wet herself. But at home she's fine. She couldn't find the toilet at the centre and I think she didn't want to ask because she felt she ought to know. I spoke to the staff and now every so often one of them takes her there.

My mother would try every door looking for the toilet, so I put a notice on the door which said 'Ladies' and she had no problem finding it. But a friend who tried this said a picture of a lavatory worked best for his mother.

Meal times

People with dementia may have poor appetite. They may not be very interested in eating. Some people with dementia seem to lose weight even when they are eating properly. They may be confused about whether they have eaten or not. Some want to start on the next meal as soon as they finish one. They may have poor table manners and become messy in their eating habits. They may have difficulty using cutlery. Eating certain foods can be a problem particularly if someone's dentures don't fit well. Too little to drink causes dehydration. This will make the person with dementia exhausted and more confused.

What you can do

1. Allow plenty of time for meals. Make sure meal times are pleasant and enjoyable.

2. Tell the person which meal it is and what there is to eat. You may have to remind the person how to eat by prompting her to pick up the fork or spoon.

3. As far as possible avoid feeding someone who has difficulty. This encourages the person to be more dependent than necessary. But sometimes spoon feeding may be needed.

4. Try not to worry too much about table manners. Allow the person to feed herself even if it is messy. Plastic table cloths are very practical.

5. If weight loss is a problem put out snacks. If the person is restless, provide tasty finger foods so that she can eat and wander at the same time.

6. See that the person gets enough to drink. She needs at least 8 cups of fluid a day. This can include soup and fruit juice as well as tea and coffee. Make sure that drinks are not too hot. Avoid too much fluid just before going to bed. If the person has dentures, check that they are in place and fit properly.

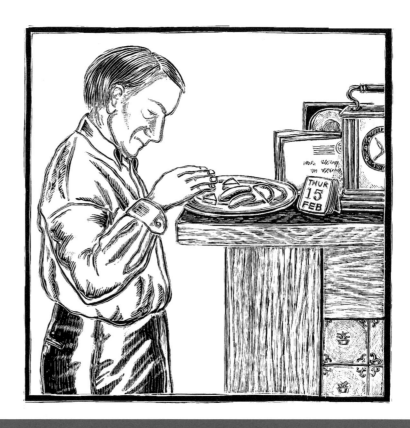

7. Ask the occupational therapist for forks and spoons that are easier to hold. If forks are difficult, the person may be happier using a spoon. You may also need to use a spill-proof cup. You can use an ordinary cup with cling film over the top and a straw inserted in it. Ask your health visitor or occupational therapist about other eating aids.

8. Try having the main meal in the middle of the day. This may help reduce night time indigestion and discomfort. It may also help the person sleep better.

10. If the person will only eat certain foods, check with the doctor that her diet is healthy.

11. For people living alone, or alone during the day, ask the social work department about meals on wheels. Try leaving out cold food such as ham, cheese, sandwiches or flasks of hot food. Don't leave cans and packets which are hard to open. However, the person may not eat food that you leave for her. If this is a problem, perhaps a home help could come in at lunch time to make sure the person eats. Ask the social work department.

12. If someone loses weight despite eating well, or seems to have lost her appetite, consult the doctor. It may be due to dementia or to another medical problem.

My partner is so restless now that he can't seem to sit and finish a meal. But he's happy to take a sandwich and eat it as he goes.

DAILY LIVING—SUMMARY

Dressing

- Allow plenty of time.
- Don't do too much for the person–encourage independence.
- Lay out clothes in the order the person is used to.
- Allow choice but you may need to limit it.
- Gently correct any errors in dressing.
- Explain what you are doing when you give help.
- If necessary, alter clothing to make dressing easier.

Appearance and personal care

- Compliment the person when she looks good.
- Remind the person about cleaning teeth or shaving.
- Show the person what to do if he gets mixed up.
- Encourage men to get used to an electric shaver early in the illness.
- Encourage the person to keep up regular dental and hair appointments.

Bathing

- Supervise bathing as required.
- Make bath-time as pleasant as you can and give reassurance.
- Use bath aids to make bathing easier and safer.
- Ask for advice and help.

Incontinence

- See the doctor first of all.
- Don't make a big issue of incontinence.
- Try occasional reminders or regular toiletting.
- Agitation may mean that the person needs to go to the toilet.
- If buttons or zips cause problems, replace them with Velcro.
- Ask your community nurse about aids.
- Make sure the person knows how to get to the toilet.
- Ensure an adequate diet.
- Get help with laundry if available.
- Restrict drinks in the evening.
- Do not use a standard electric blanket for someone who is incontinent.
- Only use laxatives if the doctor has prescribed them.

Meal times

- Allow plenty of time for eating.
- Make sure dentures fit well.
- Say what meal it is and what they will be eating.
- Buy or make eating aids.
- Be patient with untidiness.
- See that the person gets a balanced diet and enough fluid.
- Use snacks and finger foods.

- Find out about meals on wheels.
- Ask the doctor or nurse for advice.

BEHAVIOUR

Many carers find changes in the behaviour of the person they care for very difficult to handle. But there are a few basic ideas which may help. The person is more likely to feel better in a familiar environment. Try to help her feel secure. If she does something that bothers you, start by thinking about whether it is really a problem. What would happen if she did it again? Perhaps it is risky, or embarrassing. Or perhaps is it just out of the ordinary, but not harmful.

If it is a problem, you may be able to work out what is causing the behaviour. Perhaps you can avoid what starts the behaviour. If you feel there is a problem, always talk to someone about it.

The next few pages cover some of the common difficulties faced by people with dementia and their carers, and some possible solutions. No solution will work for everyone. Try different things until you find what works best.

Apathy and loss of interest

People with dementia often seem to become bored and withdrawn. They may not seem able to keep an interest in anything for more than a few minutes. This can be upsetting if you are used to seeing the person you care for busy and happy.

Some people with dementia may be depressed. This can be treated. If you think the person you care for is depressed, seek medical advice. But even without depression, apathy is common in dementia.

What you can do

1. Try to make sure that each day has something of interest for the person with dementia. It might be going for a walk, listening to favourite music, a game of cards, gardening; anything which the person enjoys.

2. Involve the person with dementia as far as possible in choosing what to do.

3. Talk about the day's activities.

4. Help the person with dementia do whatever jobs around the house she can manage. Doing these tasks can help the person to feel useful—even if you have to go over the work again later yourself!

5. Try to get other people involved. A chat with old friends, perhaps talking about the past, can help to raise the person's spirits. Old friends will soon get used to the changes in the person and make allowances.

6. Remember that a time to be quiet, sit back and do nothing can also be enjoyable.

Over the last year, my mother has found it very hard to get herself organised to do things. She tends just to sit in her chair most of the day if left to herself. But I've found that she'll enjoy doing things like sorting out the sewing box as long as I get her started.

Wandering

Many carers worry about people with dementia wandering. But remember, just because the person may not be able to tell you what she is doing doesn't mean that she is wandering aimlessly. For example, she may be looking for the toilet or have another perfectly good reason for walking about.

If you are worried about the person you care for, ask yourself first whether there is really a problem. If the person goes out, does she find the way home again? Is she able to cross the road safely? Is it a problem if she walks around the house restlessly? Perhaps the person is at risk if she goes out at night but not during the day. Or perhaps walking around the house is no problem but going out is a worry. It is important to give the person as much freedom as reasonably possible—even the freedom to take a risk sometimes.

If it *is* a problem, think about why the person may be wandering. Is she:
• bored and needing stimulation?
• setting off to do something but forgetting where she was going?
• just going for a walk, perhaps as she has always done?
• unsettled by being in a new and unfamiliar place or finding a familiar place strange?
• needing exercise?

If the person goes out at night, is she:
• mixed up about the time, not knowing whether it is day or night?
• waking up confused or frightened, not sure where know where she is?
• looking for the toilet but not able to find it?
• sleeping too much in the day-time or going to bed too early?
• in discomfort or pain for any reason?

See Further information (page 100) for more information on wandering.

What you can do

1. Keep a current photograph of the person in case she gets lost.

2. Make sure the person gets enough exercise. Try exercise to music or going out for a walk.

3. If the person is likely to get lost or be at risk outside, you may have to stop her from going out alone. Try putting a bolt at the bottom of the outside door where she may not look, as long this doesn't make her panic. Or fix a bell to the door (like a shop door bell), or windchimes, or an alarm pad under the mat, to alert you if she tries to go out.

4. If the person tends to get lost, see that she has identification such as a card, bracelet or pendant. It should show her name and a contact phone number. For security reasons, do not put her address on it.

5. If the person is lost, tell the police at once.

For day-time wandering

1. Try to find activities which will hold the person's interest. Wandering is less likely if she has something to do.

2. If the person enjoys going for a walk, it is important she can. If she is not safe alone and you can't go along, ask friends or volunteer helpers.

3. If the person with dementia insists on going to see someone who is no longer alive, it is sometimes a good idea to go along too. Gradually divert her attention to things you see or some other topic. Then suggest that it is time to go home. She may have forgotten the reason for the outing.

When he has gone to a nearby shop, and not come back, I have to go out searching. I keep my cool when I find him. Sometimes he smiles and says 'I'm glad to see you. I've had a long walk.' Other times he might refuse to get into the car so I let him go. But I keep him in sight until he's tired and agrees to take a lift home.

For night-time wandering

1. It may help if you increase day-time activity and discourage long sleeps during the day.

2. Make sure that the person has been to the toilet before going to bed.

3. If the person with dementia is restless at night, make sure she is comfortable and warm. Reassure her about where she is.

4. Leave a dim light on in the bedroom or passage to reduce confusion if the person wakes up in the dark.

5. Try to make the house as safe as possible so that you don't have to worry about the person walking around at night. For example, the occupational therapist may be able to provide an adult stair gate. Lock the kitchen door at night. Put on safe background heating.

6. The occupational therapist may be able to suggest other equipment to help, such as an alarm pad which will tell you if the person gets out of bed.

7. In some areas a night care service may be available. Check with your social work department, Crossroads, or Alzheimer Scotland—Action on Dementia. In certain circumstances the night nursing service may help—ask the doctor about this.

8. If the wandering gets out of hand, ask the doctor for a specialist assessment. Occasionally medication may help but it should not be the doctor's first thought.

My sister used to go out at all hours. I was worried because she's forgotten how to cross the road safely. I put a big notice on the inside of the door to remind her not to go out on her own, and it seems to work most times.

Attention demands and clinging

Some people with dementia want to be with their carer all the time. Someone may follow her carer from room to room, and get very distressed if the carer goes out. This may be very hard for you to bear, especially if it this reaches the point where you have no privacy.

The person with dementia may be feeling very insecure. If you leave the room, she may forget where you are or how long you have been away, so she may try to stay with you all the time.

What you can do

1. Remember that the person is feeling insecure, and offer plenty of reassurance.

2. Remember that your well-being is important. You will find it easier to cope with the person's need for attention if you get some time off.

3. Ask for help from family and friends to spend time with the person to give you a break.

4. Consider a day care or home support service (see Getting help, page 73) to give you time off.

There were times when I found it very hard indeed. She would follow me around everywhere, driving my patience to its limits. My only escape was to lock myself in the bathroom sometimes to read the paper. But now she goes to the day centre, which she loves, and I get two days a week to myself.

Anger or aggression

Some people can feel aggressive at times as a result of their dementia. Verbal abuse is more common than physical aggression. The person may shout or make accusations or threats. It can be quite a shock if a quiet and gentle person starts to be aggressive.

The person may become aggressive because she is frustrated at not being able to do things she used to be able to do. Or she may misunderstand what is going on. For example, she may put something away and forget it altogether, and then think someone else must have stolen it. Sometimes someone with dementia may over-react to something very minor. The part of the brain which would normally control her reaction may be damaged.

Some people with dementia may be aggressive only to their carers. Perhaps this is because the carer is closest to the person. Many people are more polite to strangers than to people they are close to. This may be very hard to cope with.

What you can do

1. Remain calm if you can, though this is easier said than done. Remind yourself that it is not the person's fault but the illness making her aggressive or angry. Try not to take it personally. The person will probably quickly forget the anger and upset.

2. Speak calmly and gently, and try to keep a calm and pleasant expression. Perhaps hold the person's hand. Touching someone is a good way to help her feel less isolated.

3. Remind the person what is going on around her and what will happen next and why. She is less likely to be frightened if she understands what is going on.

4. Focus on the things the person does well rather than on mistakes or failures.

5. Distract the person's attention away from the situation.

6. If the person is gripping you, try not to struggle. Stay calm and try to defuse the situation.

7. Try not to get into an argument or get angry yourself. This will only make things worse.

8. Afterwards, try to work out what caused the upset and see if there is anything you can change. For example, was she frustrated at failing to do something? If so, perhaps you can make the task easier or avoid it altogether.

9. Explain to other people, such as children or home care workers, that the anger or accusations are caused by the illness.

10. Talk to someone you trust, such as a friend, professional worker or the 24 hour Dementia Helpline. Coping with aggression, especially from someone you love, is very stressful.

11. Ask the doctor for a specialist assessment if you are worried.

12. Remember, aggression does not last for ever. Probably the person you care for will change with time and stop being aggressive.

One day I said to my Gran in a calm voice, 'Nobody in this house would steal any of your things. You can't help it because your memory isn't good, even though it can be very upsetting to who you accuse.' She agreed and repeated, 'Nobody in our family steals.' (Sarah, aged 10)

Hallucinations and delusions

Some people with dementia may hear or see things which are not there (hallucinations). Some may believe things which are not true (delusions).

More often, people with dementia may mistake what they hear or see for something else, or confuse events. For example, someone may mistake a reflection in the window for someone in the room. Or someone may think things have been stolen because she has forgotten putting them away. These may not be true hallucinations or delusions, but they can still be upsetting or frightening, and the person will need reassurance.

What you can do

1. If the person starts to get hallucinations, she should see the doctor. The problem may be caused by an infection which can be treated. Or it may be a side effect of medicines. Or the doctor may be able to prescribe medicines to stop the hallucinations.

2. If the person misunderstands what she sees, try explaining what it really is. Or change the source of the problem. There may be a simple solution. For example, turn on a light or close the curtains.

3. If the person is really hallucinating, she is experiencing something which is not there. It is pointless to tell her she is imagining it, because it is real to her. Be sympathetic and reassuring. Explain that you cannot see or hear what she can, but the you understand how she feels. Touch and comfort the person in a calm and reassuring way. This may help bring her back to reality.

4. If the person thinks someone is stealing, first check whether this is true. Just because someone has dementia does not mean she is mistaken. Someone who lives alone may be very vulnerable to people who take advantage. If you are sure that the person is deluded, talk to children, home support workers and anyone else who she may accuse of stealing to explain that this is because of her illness.

If my husband addresses remarks to someone he thinks is sitting beside him, I don't laugh or say there's no-one there. I take it calmly and say, 'Are you sure there's someone there? Is it not the pattern on the curtains?'

Embarrassing and odd behaviour

Sometimes people with dementia may do things which are embarrassing to you. The person will not realise that what she is doing is odd. For example, the person may start to use swear words at embarrassing times, or spit, or be rude to visitors. She may do things at the wrong time, such as start to undress in public.

Some embarrassing or odd behaviour may happen because the person is confused about where she is or forgets what should be done when. For some people, the illness may damage the part of the brain that controls their inhibitions, so that they just don't realise that they should not swear in company, for example.

Some things the person does may be irritating rather than embarrassing. For example, she may fidget or start to hide things.

Try to think about whether the behaviour really matters, and if so, why. Sometimes you might just learn to live with it.

What you can do

1. Explain what is happening to other people. They will usually be understanding.

2. Don't over-react. For example, if the person starts to undress in company, calmly take her to another room. Make sure that her clothes are comfortable. Check that she is not too hot or wanting to use the toilet.

3. If the person fidgets, try finding her something to do, or just try to ignore the habit. If she fidgets with clothes, try giving her a handkerchief instead.

4. If the person hides things, put important items in a safe place. In time you will get used to where she puts things. It may be a good idea to remove keys from drawers and cupboards.

5. Remember, it is the illness causing the odd behaviour, not the person doing it on purpose.

I used to get so upset when my sister ate with her fingers in company. I used to try to make her use her fork, and for a while I didn't invite anyone round. But then I thought about it, and I decided that it really didn't do anyone any harm. She wasn't worried, and my friends all said they didn't mind—it was just me being embarrassed. So I decided not to worry about it any more.

My husband was a real gentleman, but now he swears like a trooper. He isn't aggressive, he just uses words he never would have used in the presence of a lady. At first I was shocked. But now I realise he can't help it and doesn't mean it the way it sounds. He looks so surprised and hurt if I tell him off—he doesn't realise what he's doing wrong. I suppose I've learnt to live with it. I warn people before they meet him and they usually cope very well.

Sex

The person's attitude to sex and sexual relationships may change. People with dementia may sometimes lose interest in sex altogether, or want sex more often than before.

If you are caring for your partner, you may feel differently about sex too. Your relationship may have changed now that you are a carer. You may find that dressing and toileting your partner make it hard to have sexual feelings too. Your partner's personality may have changed.

You may want to carry on your sexual relationship but worry about whether you should. Some partners who continue with a sexual relationship worry that they are taking advantage of the person with dementia. You can usually tell from the person's behaviour whether this is so. Continuing a sexual relationship may help both partners feel closer.

Sex and relationships can be difficult to talk about, but try to discuss it with a friend or a professional you trust. Or you can call the Dementia Helpline confidentially and anonymously.

Sometimes someone with dementia may make a sexual approach to someone who is not his or her partner. This might be because the illness has damaged the part of the brain which controls inhibitions. Or the person might have mistaken someone for his or her partner. Or it may just be that the person wants the comfort of touch and closeness.

Any changes to do with sexual behaviour can be confusing and hard to accept.

My father sometimes thinks that I'm my mother and climbs into bed with me. The first time it happened I was very upset. I couldn't understand it. But I talked it over with the community psychiatric nurse and felt a bit better. Now when he does it I get out of bed and leave the room and then come back in saying, 'Hello Dad,' to remind him who I am without embarrassing him.

My wife and I had a very close physical relationship, but since she was diagnosed about four years ago she has gradually lost interest. It bothered me a lot at first, but we still share a bed and that helps me feel close to her. It's something I have come to accept.

What you can do

1. If you can, give the person plenty of physical contact. Hold hands, or give a hug or a cuddle.

2. If the person approaches the wrong person sexually, stay calm and try to distract and reassure him or her. Remember this is caused by the illness and is not the person's fault.

3. Talk to someone about any problems. Your doctor or your local Marriage Counselling Service or Alzheimer Scotland—Action on Dementia contact may be able to help, or be able to put you in touch with someone who can. They will not be surprised or shocked. Call the 24 hour

Dementia Helpline to talk it over confidentially. You don't need to give your name.

BEHAVIOUR—SUMMARY

Apathy and loss of interest

- Plan something of interest each day.
- Involve the person with dementia in planning as far as you can.
- Encourage the person to do tasks around the house.
- Get friends to help.
- Accept that some loss of interest is bound to happen. You don't have to fight it all the time!

Wandering

- Don't try to prevent wandering if there is no real risk.
- Keep a current photograph.
- Make sure the person gets exercise.
- You may have to stop her from going out alone.
- Give the person identification such as a card, bracelet or pendant.
- If the person is lost, tell the police at once.

For day-time wandering

- Exercise and activities may help.
- Go along too and try distraction.

For night-time wandering

- Increase day-time activity.
- Get the person to go to the toilet before going to bed.
- Make sure she is comfortable and warm and reassure her.
- Leave a dim light on.
- Try to make the house as safe as possible.
- Ask the occupational therapist about equipment.
- Ask about a night care service.
- Ask the doctor for a specialist assessment.

Attention demands and clinging

- Reassure the person.
- Arrange for breaks.

Aggression

- Keep calm.
- Try to defuse the situation.
- Distract the person.
- Don't get involved in an argument.
- Work out what triggers angry outbursts, and try to avoid it.
- Focus on successes.
- Talk about aggression problems with someone you trust
- Tell the doctor.

Hallucinations and delusions

- Get help from the doctor.
- Explain what is really there if this helps.
- Reassure the person.
- Look for practical solutions such as closing the curtain.
- Explain the situation to others.

Embarrassing and odd behaviour

- This is caused by the illness. Explain this to others.
- Deal with the situation in a matter-of-fact way.
- Learn what odd behaviour is likely and try to avoid it.
- If the person tends to lose or hide things, remove important items to a secure place.

Sex

- Discuss problems with someone you trust.

RISKS AND HAZARDS

Safety in the home

Dementia increases the chance of accidents. It is hard for carers to know how far they should go in trying to protect the person with dementia (or others) from possible risks. It is worth taking a few simple steps to prevent accidents. But you cannot remove all dangers. You can't avoid a certain degree of risk if the person is to keep some independence. If you don't live with the person you care for, safety can be a particular worry.

Try to assess what the real risks are. Observe what the person can and can't do. For example, can she use a gas fire safely? If there is a danger, such as a burning pan, does she react appropriately or not? The booklet *Keeping Safe: a guide to safety when someone with dementia lives alone* gives more information on risk and safety—see Further information. The occupational therapist will be able to tell you about the safety aids mentioned below.

What you can do

1. Check the home for anything which might cause a fall. Repair or secure any loose banister rails, slippery floor mats and loose carpet edges. Check for badly placed furniture.

2. Electrical appliances and plugs need to be checked regularly. Make sure that cables and wires do not trail across floors. If the person is incontinent don't let her use an ordinary electric blanket.

3. Check that bright enough lights are used throughout the house. Use night lights to help the person find the way about at night.
4. Fit smoke alarms and make sure neighbours know they are there.

5. The lighting of steps and stairs is very important. You can paint the edge of outside steps with a white line to make it easily seen. An extra hand rail on the stairs can be very helpful.

6. Have hand rails fitted on the bath and by the toilet and put a non-slip mat in the bath or shower.

7. Use a guard in front of any fire. The large nursery type is best, hooked on to the wall or fireplace.

8. Gas appliances should be checked for leaks. British Gas has a Gas Care Register for people who are disabled or over 60 and living alone or with other people over 60. This gives the right to a free safety check every three years.

9. Keep cleaning fluids, bleach, paints, and so on out of reach. Some people with dementia may think they are ordinary drinks.

10. If the person cooks or lights a fire, make sure she can still do this safely. Put large clear instructions beside the appliance. If the person cannot use appliances safely make sure that she only uses them when someone is there. Using only one gas ring lessens the danger. British Gas can arrange this. An automatic electric kettle may be useful if the person can learn to use it.

11. If the person becomes unsafe with a gas fire, it may be better replaced. Some carers recommend an oil-filled electric radiator or an electric heater on a timer switch.

My father's neighbour was worried about him using his gas cooker because a couple of times he forgot to light it. But he didn't want to stop cooking. I talked to the gas board, who fitted a gas isolation tap. Now he cooks his lunch while his home help is there, and she turns the gas off when she leaves.

Driving

Most people with dementia will not be safe to drive. However, some people who are diagnosed very early on in the illness may continue to drive safely for a while. Ask the person's specialist doctor to assess whether she is still safe to drive. You must tell the insurance company and the DVLC about a diagnosis of dementia.

If the person is not safe you will have to persuade her to give up driving. Ask the doctor's advice on this. It is a difficult issue but don't wait until there is an accident.

What you can do

1. If possible encourage the person to get used to other transport such as buses and trains early on in the illness.

2. Raise the subject of driving tactfully. Point out the hazards. If possible, also point out the benefits of not having to drive.

3. If the person does not want to stop driving, ask other carers how they handled the problem.

4. The person may find it easier to accept that she must stop driving if someone in authority says so. Ask the doctor or the police to help.

5. Make other arrangements for transport. Try to make up a rota of drivers or suggest using buses. Some groups such as the WRVS may be able to help with transport. Check with the social work department, as some local councils have taxi schemes for disabled people.

My mother used to rely on her car and didn't want to stop driving. But I could see that she wasn't really safe any more. I talked to her about it, but in the end it was the doctor who told her she'd have to stop. He said she should think of it as if she was finding it hard to see properly.

I tried to get my husband to stop driving but he just wouldn't be told. I was worried in the car with him. I had to remind him which way to go round roundabouts. I hid the car keys but he got angry and threatened me. In the end my son took a vital bit out of the engine, so the car wouldn't start. He was frustrated for a while but at least he didn't blame me.

Smoking and alcohol

Smoking and drinking cause problems in dementia. Smoking is a fire hazard for people who are forgetful. A drink or two causes slight loss of mental alertness in anyone. For a person with dementia such a loss has greater effects and could increase confusion. The occasional drink in company is not always a bad idea. However, care and supervision are needed. Risks may arise when someone is on medication and has a drink.

What you can do

1. Try to persuade the person with dementia to stop smoking or cut down. Many people with dementia forget to smoke and then do not miss the habit once it is broken.

2. If the person continues to smoke make sure she does not abandon lighted cigarettes or throw them away in waste paper baskets. Stop the person from smoking in bed.

3. Put big ashtrays everywhere. Put an ashtray at hand height beside the person's favourite chair. Replace wastepaper baskets with metal bins.

4. Fit smoke alarms in all rooms.

5. Keep matches out of reach.

6. Buy flame resistant clothes and furniture.

7. If the person is using nicotine patches make sure she does not smoke, as this greatly increases the health risks.

8. Don't leave alcohol where the person with dementia can help herself. The person may not remember how much she has had. You may have to lock alcohol up or hide it.

9. Ask the doctor's advice about whether the person can have any alcoholic drink and, if so, how much. This is essential if the person is taking medicines.

My brother has always liked a few drinks, but he started forgetting how many he'd had and drinking far too much. My sister and I do his shopping now, so we bought some low alcohol lager to see if he'd like it. He still gets through a lot of cans—but at least he doesn't get drunk now!

Medicines

You will have to take special care if the person with dementia is on any sort of medicine. She may forget how many tablets she has had. She may accidentally take too many or not take them at all. Check with the doctor to make sure the person is only taking what is necessary.

What you can do

1. Ask the doctor if each medicine is really necessary. If it is, ask if it the person can take it in a simpler way, such as once a day instead of three times.

2. Do not leave it to the person with dementia to see to medication. She is likely to forget or to take too much. It is better if one person is in charge of medicines.

3. If you can't supervise medication completely, there are several ideas which might help. You can leave the right daily dose in containers. Ask the pharmacist about special containers with compartments for each dose. A clearly printed note about when to take each item may help early on in the illness.

4. Keep all medicine bottles clearly labelled and in a locked medicine cupboard.

5. Keep a weekly or monthly record sheet on the inside of the medicine cupboard. Note on the sheet which tablets the person should take each day. When you give a tablet, mark the record sheet to show that you have given it. This helps to stop mistakes, especially if more than one person is involved.

6. Make sure that you are clear about which medicine to give when. If not, check with the doctor.

7. Make sure that both the hospital doctor and the GP know about all the drugs being taken. Even medicines bought over the counter, such as laxatives or aspirin, can cause problems when taken with other medicines.

8. Make a note of any side effects and let the doctor know.

9. Get rid of medicines not in use. The safest way to do this is to take them to the chemist.

When I looked in my father-in-law's medicine cabinet I found almost twenty different prescription drugs. Some dated back more than five years. I checked with his doctor and he was only on one pill three times a day. So I took the rest to the chemist's to be disposed of.

RISKS AND HAZARDS—SUMMARY

Safety in the home

- Check for risks and make repairs as needed.
- Fit smoke alarms.
- Make sure lights are bright enough.
- Use fire guards.
- Keep bleach, paints, and so on out of reach.
- Make sure that the person can use heaters and cookers safely.
- Ask for advice from British Gas, Scottish Power or Hydro-Electric.
- Remember that you can't prevent all risks. The person needs freedom too.
- Ask an occupational therapist about safety.

Driving

- Ask the doctor if the person is safe to drive.
- Tell the insurance company and the DVLC of the person's diagnosis.
- Discuss with the person with dementia when driving should stop.
- Consider other ways to travel.

Smoking and alcohol

- Try to persuade the person with dementia to stop smoking.
- Keep matches out of reach.
- Put big ashtrays everywhere.
- Fit smoke alarms.
- Don't leave alcohol where the person can drink unsupervised.
- Ask the doctor whether the person can drink alcohol.

Medicines

• Ask the doctor if medicines are necessary and given as simply as possible.

• Don't leave the person to take medicines alone.

• Work out a system for making sure that the person takes the right medicine at the right time.

• Watch for side effects and inform the doctor.

• Make sure that the doctor knows about all medicines the person is taking.

• Get rid of medicines not in use.

Section 5
GETTING HELP

Dementia does not only affect the person with the illness. It affects family and friends too. Caring for someone with dementia can affect your social life, work, leisure time, financial situation and family relationships.

Don't try to cope on your own. Remember, to go on caring for as long as you want to you must look after yourself too. There are many different services which can support you and the person you look after. This section describes some of the services you may find helpful and how to find them. It also lists professionals who can help people with dementia and their carers. When you talk to a professional, don't be tempted to make a good impression or say things are all right when they are not. He or she needs to know how things really are to help you.

The help you need will change during the course of the person's illness. At the beginning, you may need information and help coming to terms with the illness and making plans. Later you may need time off, and the person with dementia may benefit from the stimulation of a day centre, for example.

To get practical services, talk to the social work department about community care services and to the person's family doctor or community nurse about health services.

MAKE A PLAN

To start planning what help you could use, you might find it useful to make a list.
• What problems face you and the person you care for?
• What do you want to know?
• What do you and the person with dementia need for practical help and emotional support?

The national 24 hour Dementia Helpline on 0800 317 817 is a good place to start. They can help you work out what help might be useful and can put you in touch with services near you. Alzheimer Scotland—Action on Dementia and other organisations have produced free guides to local services for many parts of Scotland. Ask the Dementia Helpline if there is one for your area.

COMMUNITY CARE

Both the person with dementia and you, as a carer, have a right to a community care assessment. Call your local social work department to ask for an assessment. They will arrange for a social worker or another community care professional to visit and talk to the person with dementia and to the carer. If you agree, the worker doing the assessment will talk also to other people with relevant information, such as the doctor. He or she should assess the needs of the person with dementia and of the carer separately. Assessment is free, but you may have to pay something for any services (see Charges for care services, page 76).

If the assessment shows that you or the person with dementia need services, the person doing the assessment will put together a care plan. The care plan will set out details of a 'package of care', using local services to try to meet your needs. You should be given a copy of the care plan. The services may be provided by the social work department or by voluntary or private organisations.

Sometimes there is a waiting list for assessments. If you need help right away, ask the social work department if they can do an emergency assessment.

My mother is very good at being polite and sociable. She thinks she does all her own cooking and shopping, but in fact I do everything. But she gets very anxious and confused when I'm not with her. When the social worker came to assess my mother I was worried he wouldn't see the true picture. So I asked him to stay with my mother for ten minutes while I nipped out to the shops. When I came back he said, 'I don't know how you've been coping.'

Help at home

Home care services (sometimes called domiciliary services) can offer care for the person with dementia in her own home, depending on what she needs. For example, a home help might help the person to prepare a meal, or a care assistant might help her to get dressed or go out for a walk. For many carers, this gives the freedom of a few hours without worry. Home care services can also help people with dementia who live alone to cope and to live at home safely for as long as they can. In some areas, overnight home care services may be available to enable a carer to get a good night's sleep. Ask the social work department or call the Dementia Helpline for details of services in your area.

Home helps

Home helps are provided by the social work department. In many areas, home helps are now providing personal care services more than, for example, doing the cleaning. Often they also provide much-needed company.

Home support services

Some voluntary organisations provide home care or 'sitter' services. For example, Crossroads runs schemes in many areas, providing trained care assistants to help look after the person with dementia. They do more than just 'sit' with the person. They may provide stimulating activities or outings, for example.

Private nursing or care agencies can also provide care assistants or nurses during the day or at night. You will have to pay for this. You can find them in the local Yellow Pages.

Day centres

A place at a day centre can give the person with dementia a chance to socialise and to enjoy stimulating activities. It will also give you some time off. Most day centres will arrange transport. Evening and weekend care are also available in some areas. Some day centres are run by the social work department, others by voluntary organisations such as Alzheimer Scotland—Action on Dementia.

Some people with mild dementia attend day centres which cater for elderly people; others need specialist dementia day care. Specialist day centres provide activities suited to the person's abilities. They can often cater even for people whose dementia is quite severe.

My husband didn't want to go to the day centre at all. Although he's 81, he hated the idea of 'sitting around with all those old people'. But I persuaded him to try it and went with him the first couple of times and now he loves it. They go on outings, and he gets a game of snooker with one of the volunteers most days. Now he goes twice a week and I get the peace and quiet I need to help me cope.

In some areas there are now day centres particularly for younger people with dementia. But in many areas younger people go to day centres which cater mostly for older people. If you care for a younger person, ask the social work department about services in your area. If they are not appropriate, you may want to ask the social work department to develop specialist services.

Respite breaks

Everyone needs time off sometimes. Caring for someone with dementia can be a tiring and often stressful job. A respite break, when the person with dementia goes into a residential or nursing home, or sometimes a hospital, will

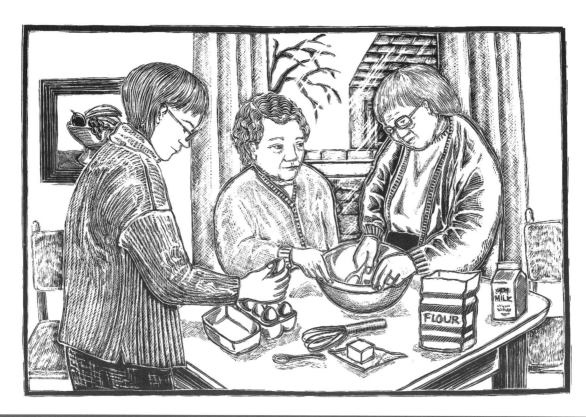

give you the chance to recharge your batteries. Perhaps you might take a holiday, or maybe just have some time for yourself at home.

I felt very guilty about letting my father go into respite care for a fortnight. Last time he went he came back more confused because of the change of environment, although the home said he was fine while he was there. But when I talked it over at the carers' group they pointed out that I must look after myself if I want to go on looking after him for as long as I can.

There are three routes to respite.

Respite through the social work department

If you are assessed as needing respite, the social worker or care manager should try to arrange a place in a residential or nursing home. The type of home depends on what is suitable for the person you care for. If you haven't been assessed as needing respite, but you feel you need a break, call the social work department and ask for a new assessment. There may be a charge for respite care. The amount depends on where you live and on your income and capital.

Private respite

Some residential and nursing homes offer respite places. If you arrange this privately, you will have to pay the home's fees. Make sure the home you choose is suitable. Visit, preferably with the person you care for, talk to the staff and if you can, talk to residents and their relatives.

Respite through the health service

In some areas, the GP or hospital specialist can sometimes arrange a respite place in hospital. There is no charge for this.

Holidays

Both you and the person with dementia may enjoy a holiday, either together or separately. Many people with dementia manage very well in hotels or guest houses, but for information on other places which are suitable for people with dementia, call the Dementia Helpline. Alzheimer Scotland—Action on Dementia has a holiday home in Edinburgh for people with dementia and carers.

Laundry service

Some areas have a laundry service for people who have extra washing because of continence problems. Ask the social work department or the district nurse.

Meals services

Meals on Wheels and other similar services can provide a hot meal delivered to the person's house. Ask the social work department about the service.

Charges for care services

Each social work department has different charges for services such as day care, home care or respite. The social worker or care manager will do a financial assessment to work out how much someone can afford to pay. The amount depends on the income and individual circumstances of the person with dementia. Many people pay nothing at all or only a small amount.

If the person does not want the service

Someone with dementia may not want to accept a service for a number of reasons. Perhaps the person thinks she is coping perfectly well, and doesn't realise the need for help. Perhaps she is reluctant to have a stranger in the house. Or she may have negative ideas about day centres. She may not want to go into respite care for fear of being taken away from home. Often this is more of a problem earlier in the illness The person may feel that independence is being taken away. Later, she may be more willing to agree.

What you can do

1. Talk to the person with dementia about the service you think might help. Try to explain why you think it is a good idea, and how the service will help both of you.

2. Talk to the social worker, nurse or someone else for advice.

3. Suggest a trial period. The person may well find that she enjoys a day centre, for example.

4. Offer to go with the person to a day centre for the first few visits, or to be there when a home care worker comes.

5. Reassure her that respite is just for a holiday and that she will be coming home.

My wife hated the idea of going into respite and I put it off for a long time. But I was making myself ill, getting up with her two or three times a night. Eventually I told her that I needed the break and she agreed to go just for the weekend. When she came back from the residential home she wanted to know how soon she could go back to 'that lovely hotel'!

Community care rights

Under the Community Care Act, everyone who needs it has a right to a community care assessment. However, the social work department does not have to provide any of the services this assessment says the person needs, although they will normally try to. Sometimes it may take time to get the services you feel you need.

However, the social work department must also assess someone under the Chronically Sick and Disabled Persons Act 1970 when they are doing a community care assessment for a disabled person. This includes most people with dementia. If they assess someone as needing certain services this Act says they *must* offer those services. These services are:
• help at home
• recreational or leisure facilities
• a telephone
• transport
• home adaptations
• a holiday
• meals.

If the social work department wants to stop one of these services, they should reassess the person first. Aspects of these arrangements are currently under review. If the social work department wants to cut one of these services for the person you care for, call the Dementia Helpline for up-to-date information.

If you are not satisfied

The social work department will usually try to provide a service. But sometimes you may not agree with what they think you and the person need. Or you may be told the person can't have a service because there is no space, or because the social work department has other priorities. If you are not satisfied, ask for a review of the assessment or the care plan. The social work department should look again at the assessment and the care plan and may agree to make changes.

If you are still not satisfied you may make a complaint. There is no right of appeal in community care law. But every social work department must by law have a complaints procedure. Ask them for information on how to make a complaint. You can get help with making a complaint from the Dementia Helpline.

If your complaint is not upheld, you may be able to go to the local authority ombudsman or take legal action. A lawyer may be able to help you seek a judicial review of the social work department's decision.

You can of course make comments to the social work department as well as complaints. You may wish to point out gaps in services which you feel should be given priority.

HEALTH SERVICES FOR PEOPLE WITH DEMENTIA

Diagnosis

A proper diagnosis is very important (see page 3). The person's general practitioner (GP) or family doctor may make the diagnosis. Or the doctor may refer the person to a hospital specialist. She would see a psychiatrist or neurologist (if she is under 65) or an old age psychiatrist (if she is over 65). The person is entitled to ask to be referred to a specialist. The specialist may visit at home or see the person at a clinic. The GP or specialist can also arrange for other health services such as a day hospital or an assessment in hospital.

If you are concerned about the person you care for, you can talk to her doctor. Make an appointment. If you have a lot to discuss, ask for a double appointment or a time at the end of a surgery so that you don't feel rushed. Make a list before you go so that you remember everything you want to say. The doctor may not be able to tell you about the person's health without her permission because of confidentiality. But your information will help, especially when the person does not have a clear idea of her own problems.

If you can, talk to the person you care for before you visit the doctor. If the person tells the doctor she wants you as her patient's supporter, you can be with her when she sees the doctor, and the doctor can give you information about her health.

Alzheimer Scotland—Action on Dementia publish a useful booklet called *Getting Help From Your Doctor* (see Further information).

General health care

The GP will also look after the person's general health. It is important to tell the doctor at once if there is a sudden change. Don't just assume that any change is due to dementia. For example, if the person seems suddenly more confused she may have an infection. If this is treated, the confusion may get better.

By law, the GP must offer to see every patient over 75 once a year or arrange for another health professional to do this.

Assessment units

The doctor may arrange for the person to go into an assessment unit in the hospital for a few weeks. The person can be given special diagnostic tests if they are necessary. Or the unit may try to help a particularly troubling problem such as hallucinations or aggression. The person may see an occupational therapist or hospital social worker.

Day hospital

The person with dementia may be offered a place at a day hospital. At the day hospital, she can be medically assessed. The day hospital may offer services such as occupational therapy assessment, nursing assessment, physiotherapy, bathing or chiropody. The person with dementia will be able to take part in stimulating activities. A place at a day hospital for the person you care for will also give you some time off. Day hospitals do not usually offer longer term support. They may refer the person on to a day centre.

If you are not satisfied with the GP or hospital service

If you are not happy with the GP's diagnosis or with the service he or she gives, you can:
• discuss your concerns with the GP
• ask the GP for a second opinion from a specialist
• make a complaint by speaking or writing to the GP practice or the health board
• change GP by asking another GP to put you on his or her list.

If you are unhappy with a hospital service, you can:
• speak to the person in charge
• make a written complaint to the unit general manager or the chief executive of the NHS trust which runs the hospital.

Every part of the national health service has a complaints procedure. If you need to you can ask for information on how to make a complaint. If you are not happy with the outcome of your complaint, you can ask for an independent review.

INFORMATION AND SUPPORT

Dementia Helpline

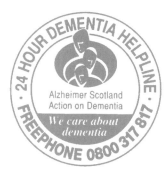

The 24 hour Dementia Helpline is on 0800 317 817. Calls are free. The Helpline is answered by trained staff and volunteers, many of whom have been carers themselves. They can give information on anything to do with dementia, from how to cope with particular problems to where to find services locally. The also offer emotional support. You can talk over your feelings or use the Helpline as a shoulder to cry on, day or night, 365 days a year. Your call is confidential and you don't even have to give your name.

Carers' support groups

A carers' support group gives you the chance to meet other people who also care for someone, for emotional support and good ideas and tips on coping. Many carers' support groups also have guest speakers who are a very useful source of information. Ask the Dementia Helpline or the social work department about groups near you.

Advocacy

Some areas have independent advocacy services. They offer advice and support for people with dementia who need help to make sure their views are heard. Ask the social work department or the Dementia Helpline.

Health education

Your local health promotion office can provide leaflets, videos and information on local support groups. They can also provide information on conferences. Find them in the 'phone book listed under the health board.

Carer's emergency card

You may be worried about what would happen to the person you look after if you were in an accident or taken ill. If so, carry a note of who to contact in an emergency. Some organisations, such as the Carers National Association produce a special card you can fill in with details of who you care for.

VOLUNTARY ORGANISATIONS

Many voluntary organisations can help you care for the person with dementia. Some, like Alzheimer Scotland—Action on Dementia, Crossroads or Age Concern Scotland, and many small local organisations, may provide services such as day care or home support. They may provide information, someone to talk to or carers' groups. See Further information for more details on individual voluntary organisations.

THE PEOPLE WHO HELP

Different social work departments and health boards organise services in different ways. In some areas staff will work in teams, and there may be an overlap in what they do. For example, in some areas, community care assessments are usually done by social workers. In other areas they may be done by occupational therapists, community psychiatric nurses or other professionals as well as social workers. However, this section will give you an idea of what each person specialises in.

Social worker

The social worker will often be the person who visits and assesses the needs of the person with dementia and of the carer. He or she should know what services are available locally. For example, if the person with dementia needs day care, the social worker will try to find a place at a suitable day centre. Social workers can help you find help with problems, both practical and to do with emotions or relationships. They can be a source of advice and support for the family.

Care manager

Care managers work for the social work department. The care manager's job is to organise a 'package of care' for someone who needs a lot of help.

My mother's care manager found her a place at a day centre for three days and one evening a week, plus a sitter service every Saturday morning and one evening a fortnight. She goes into respite for a week every three months too. It means that I can work part time and get some time with my family, while still caring for her.

Family doctor

The family doctor or general practitioner (GP) can be a very good source of help and information. He or she can help make sure the person with dementia stays as physically healthy as possible. He or she can put you in touch with other health professionals such as community nurses, physiotherapists, health visitors and hospital services.

Old age psychiatrist

People who are over 65 and have dementia, or have memory problems but have not been diagnosed may be referred to an old age psychiatrist (or psychogeriatrician) at a local hospital. Old age psychiatrists are doctors who specialise in the physical and mental health needs of older people.

If you would like the person you care for to see an old age psychiatrist, ask the GP to refer her. Patients have a right to ask for a second opinion.

Psychiatrist or neurologist

People who are under 65 and have dementia, or have memory problems but have not yet been diagnosed may be referred to a psychiatrist or a neurologist at a local hospital. Psychiatrists are doctors who specialise in mental health, including dementia. Neurologists specialise in illnesses of the brain.

If you would like the person you care for to see a specialist, ask the GP to refer her. Patients have a right to a second opinion.

Community psychiatric nurse

The community psychiatric nurse (CPN) can give emotional support to help both carers and people with dementia after a diagnosis of dementia and throughout the illness. They may be able to visit regularly. They also offer information about the illness and on practical ways of coping with the illness and the problems it can bring. They should know what services are available locally to help.

District or community nurse

The district or community nurse can visit and assess and advise on the nursing needs of the person with dementia, such as bathing or incontinence. Ask the GP or contact the community nursing service directly. In most areas they are based at the health centre or GP's surgery.

Practice nurse

The practice nurse is based at the GP surgery and can give help and advice on health problems.

Health visitor

A health visitor can assess and advise or any problems related to health. Contact the health visitor at the health centre or GP surgery.

Occupational therapist

The occupational therapist (OT) is expert at helping people to continue doing as much as they can in their daily lives. An OT can visit the person at home to assess risk and suggest ways to improve safety and to maintain independence. He or she can recommend the right equipment to help, from bath and toilet aids to memory aids. You might be able to borrow equipment to try it out. You can find an OT through the social work department or through the hospital psychiatric service.

Clinical psychologist

A clinical psychologist can work with people with dementia to help them learn ways of overcoming difficulties or coping better. He or she may be able to help someone find ways to get around memory problems, for example. The psychologist may be able to help people in the early stages of dementia to overcome feelings of anxiety or depression.

The clinical psychologist can help carers deal with stress and feelings such as grief. He or she may be able to help with specific behaviour problems such as aggression, wandering and self-care problems.

Clinical psychologists are usually based in hospitals. Ask the GP or a dementia team member if you would like to see a clinical psychologist.

Chiropodist

Chiropodists usually work in clinics, but can make home visits. Chiropody is free to retired people. Ask your doctor or the chiropody department of your local health board for details.

Dentist

Some dentists will do home visits. Talk to the person's dentist about this or ask your local health board about the Community Dental Service.

GETTING HELP—SUMMARY

Community care services

The social work department can arrange:
• Community care assessments for you and the person with dementia.
• Care management
• Home care services (sometimes called domiciliary services).
• Day centres.
• Respite breaks.
• Holidays.
• Laundry service.
• Meals services.
• Community occupational therapists.
• Residential or nursing home places.

Health services

The National Health Service provides:
• Diagnosis by the person's general practitioner (GP) or hospital specialist.

- General health care by the GP.
- Help with diagnosis or troubling problems at a hospital assessment unit.
- Day hospitals.
- Occupational therapists at day hospitals.
- Dentists.
- Psychologists.
- Chiropodists.
- Physiotherapists.
- Community psychiatric nurses.
- District or community nurses.
- Practice nurses.
- Health visitors.
- Respite in hospital.

Information and support

You can find information and support from:
- The 24 hour Dementia Helpline on 0800 317 817 can tell you about services near you.
- Local branches of Alzheimer Scotland—Action on Dementia and other voluntary organisations.
- Carers' support groups.
- Advocacy projects.
- Health promotion departments.
- NHS Helpline 0800 22 44 88

LONG-STAY CARE

Eventually, you may not be able to go on looking after the person with dementia at home. Perhaps she has become too ill for you to cope. Or perhaps your own health has changed. Not everyone can be a carer and it is important to understand and accept what you can and can't do.

COPING WITH YOUR FEELINGS

It may be very hard for you to accept that you can no longer care for the person with dementia. You may feel guilty or think that other people will disapprove. It may be hard to know what you will do with all the spare time you suddenly have. You may feel lonely without the person you were looking after and feel a sense of loss.

It is probably impossible to avoid these feelings. It may help to talk to friends or professional about how you feel, or to call the Dementia Helpline. In time you will probably realise that your decision is for the best. It can be a comfort to see the person settle in and enjoy your visits. Taking the person out for a walk, a run in the car, or a day at home may still be possible. You may also be able to help with personal care.

Admitting to myself that I couldn't go on looking after my partner was very hard. I now realise I struggled on far too long because I felt so bad about letting other people care for her. But now she's in a nursing home quite nearby and she's getting better care than I could manage on my own. And I feel much more relaxed. I visit her often and because I no longer have to do all the routine tasks I find I enjoy our time together much more.

TYPES OF LONG-TERM CARE

The type of long-term care will depend on what the person with dementia needs.

Most people with dementia who need long-term care will go into a residential home or a nursing home.

A residential home is suitable if the person needs some help or supervision but does not need nursing care. Residential homes are run by the social work department, private companies or voluntary organisations. They are all registered and inspected by the social work department.

A nursing home is suitable if the person needs nursing care. Nursing homes are usually run by private companies. They are registered and inspected by the health board. Some nursing homes specialise in looking after people with dementia.

Some people with dementia may need to go into a long-stay hospital ward. This would be arranged by the psychiatrist or old age psychiatrist. Usually only people who have quite severe dementia and problems with behaviour and who can't be cared for in a nursing home go into hospital. There is no charge for NHS hospital care.

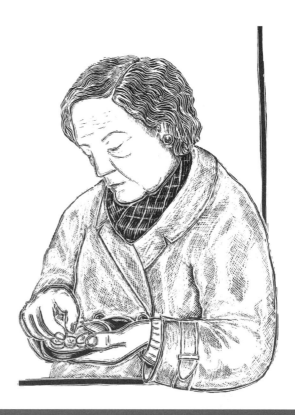

ARRANGING AND PAYING FOR LONG-TERM CARE

Residential and nursing home fees can cost hundreds of pounds a week. If the person with dementia has enough income to pay the fees, you can arrange a place in a home yourself. Ask the social work department and the health board for lists. It is a good idea to talk to the doctor or social worker first to make sure that you choose a suitable home. You may want to talk to other carers or to professionals about what each home is like.

Many people will need some help with paying nursing or residential home fees. If the person is likely to need help, either now or in the future, consult the social work department. They will assess the person if going into a residential or nursing home is the right choice for her.

If the social work department agrees that the person needs nursing or residential home care and needs help to pay for it, they should find a suitable place. If you prefer somewhere else, the social work department may agree as long as it is suitable and costs the same or less. If it costs more, you or someone else could agree to pay the extra. But if you stop paying the person may have to move.

The social work department will also give the person a financial assessment. They will look at the person's income and capital. The person's income will be used to pay the home fees. She should always be left with a weekly personal allowance (at least £13.75 from April 1996). If the person's income is not enough to pay the full fees, the social work department may help. From 1 April 1996, if the person has savings (capital) or property worth more than £16,000, she will have to pay the home fees until the amount reduces to £16,000. If the person has between £16,000 and £10,000, she will have to pay part of the fees. If she has less than £10,000, the social work department will pay, up to their maximum amount.

The house

If the person owns a house the social work department will normally count it as part of her capital. But the social work department must ignore it if one of these people still lives there:

• person's husband or wife, or unmarried heterosexual partner

• a relative who is over 60 or incapacitated

• a child under 16.

The social work department can also decide to ignore the value of the house if someone else still lives there, such as a carer. Seek advice from the Dementia Helpline or a lawyer if you live with the person with dementia and the social work department say they will take the house into account.

IF YOU ARE NOT SATISFIED WITH THE HOME

If you are not satisfied about the person's care at the residential or nursing home, you can make a complaint. All residential care and nursing homes should have a complaints policy. They should give you information about it if you ask.

First of all, speak or write to the person in charge of the home. If you are still not satisfied, you can write to the authority which registers and inspects the home. For residential homes, write to the head of the Registration and Inspection Service at your local council. For nursing homes, write to the head of the Registration and Inspection Unit at the health board.

FEELINGS OF LOSS

Some carers say that dementia itself is like a long slow bereavement. You may feel that you are gradually losing the person you once knew. Many carers feel a great sense of loss when the person is admitted to hospital or a residential or nursing home for long-stay care. Even when it is obvious that the person needs to move, some carers feel guilty at handing over much of the task of caring.

Because of the 'slow bereavement' of dementia, many people find sorrow when the person dies is mixed with relief that so much suffering is over. Some people feel less sad than they feel they should because they have already done so much grieving.

It takes time, of course, to come to terms with bereavement. At first most of your memories of the person with dementia may be about the years of the illness. In time you begin to remember her before the illness. This can be a comfort. You may find that feelings of stress and emotional upset stay for quite some time.

This is when you may appreciate the help of family and old friends. Keep in touch with other carers too. They can help you come to terms with your feelings.

If you have been the main carer it will leave a big gap in your life if the person goes into long-stay care or dies. But eventually you will begin to pick up the threads of your own life again.

When my mother died after ten years of Alzheimer's disease, she was very different from her real self. In a way I felt I started to lose her long before she actually passed on. But she still left a huge gap in my life. It's now two years since her death, and I have managed to pick up the pieces of my own life again. Even though I will always miss her, the worst feelings are past now and I find I can remember her as she used to be before she got ill.

LONG STAY CARE—SUMMARY

• Talk to friends or professionals about how you feel.
• The type of long-term care will depend on what the person with dementia needs.
• Talk to the social work department about homes and help with paying fees.

Section 7
FURTHER INFORMATION

USEFUL ORGANISATIONS

Alzheimer Scotland—Action on Dementia

8 Hill Street, Edinburgh EH2 3JZ
Office: 0131-225 1453; 24 hour Dementia
Helpline: 0800 317 817 (freephone)

Helps people with dementia, their carers and families.
Aims to be the national voice of people with dementia and
their carers and works to improve public policies.
Publishes reports, information leaflets and booklets.
Provides services around Scotland, including information,
day care, home support, befriending, advocacy, carers'
education, carers' support groups and the national 24 hour
Dementia Helpline. Call the Dementia Helpline for a free
information pack for carers or a publications list.

Alzheimer's Disease Society

Gordon House, 10 Greencoat Place,
London SW1P 1PH 0171-306 0606

Works to help people with dementia and their carers in
England, Wales and Northern Ireland. It provides
information and publications and works to improve public
policy. Local branches provide services such as day care
and home support. Ask for a publications list.

Age Concern Scotland

113 Rose Street, Edinburgh EH2 3DT 0131-220 3345

Aims to improve the quality of life for older people in
Scotland. Supports a network of over 400 local groups and
organisations. Provides advisory, information and training
services for all concerned with older people. Send stamped
addressed envelope for publications list.

Carers National Association

11 Queen's Crescent, Glasgow G4 9AS 0141-333 9495

A UK-wide organisation which campaigns and lobbies on
behalf of all carers. Provides an information and advice
service for carers and those interested in carers' issues. In
addition to a direct information service, provides
consultancy and support to a wide variety of carers'
initiatives across Scotland.

Citizens Advice Scotland

26 George Square, Edinburgh EH8 9LD 0131-667 0156

For details of your nearest Citizens Advice Bureau.

Crossroads Care Attendant Scheme

Scottish Headquarters, 24 George Square,
Glasgow G2 1EG 0141-226 3793

Local Crossroads branches provide trained care workers for home support.

Cruse Bereavement Care

18 South Trinity Road Edinburgh, EH5 3PN
0131-551 1511

Provides bereavement counselling and support groups. Call for details of local contacts.

Dementia Helpline

0800 317 817 freephone, 24 hours

Trained volunteers provide information and emotional support to carers and people with dementia. Information is available on any subject to do with dementia, from where to find help to legal and financial matters. Run by Alzheimer Scotland—Action on Dementia.

Disability Scotland

Princes House, 5 Shandwick Place, Edinburgh EH2 4RG
0131-229 8632

Provides an information service including a database of aids and equipment.

Dementia Services Development Centre

University of Stirling, Stirling, FK9 4LA 01786 467740

Exists to extend and improve services for people with dementia and their carers. Provides information, development assistance, publications, research, training, conferences and seminars for managers, planners and providers of services in the statutory, voluntary and private sectors. Ask for a publications list or a training events brochure.

Help the Aged Seniorline

0800 65 00 65 freephone, 10 a.m. to 4 p.m. Monday to Friday

Information and advice for senior citizens, their relatives, carers and friends. Information available on welfare benefits, housing, health services, support for carers, care in the community residential and nursing homes, equipment and adaptations, insurance and sources of local help.

Legal Services Agency Mental Health Legal Representation Projects (Strathclyde and Lothian)

11th Floor, Fleming House, 134 Renfrew Street, Glasgow G3 6ST 0141-353 3354
and 18 Walker Street, Edinburgh EH3 7LP 0131-225 2343

Qualified solicitors give free and confidential advice on all aspects of the law relating to dementia. Legal representation is also available; there may be a charge for this, but you may be able to get Legal Aid.

Pet Fostering Service Scotland

0141-332 7910

Call for details of your local organiser. Organises volunteers to care for pets in an emergency.

PUBLICATIONS

The 36 Hour Day: a family guide to caring at home for people with Alzheimer's disease and other confusional illnesses by Nancy L. Mace and Peter V. Rabins, MD with Beverley A. Castleton, Evelyn McEwen and Barbara Meredith, Hodder and Stoughton, co-published with Age Concern, 0-340-56382-6, £9.99

Aimed at carers, this is a useful and clearly-written book which covers most aspects of caring.

Activities and Activities II, Carole Archibald, Dementia Services Development Centre, £5.00 and £7.50 (or £10.00 for both)

Useful suggestions on suitable failure-free activities for people with dementia.

Aggression by Graham Stokes, Winslow Press, 0-86388-055-X, £8.55

Practical guidance on coping with aggressive behaviour.

The Care Maze: the law and your rights to community care in Scotland by Colin McKay and Hilary Patrick, Enable and Scottish Association for Mental Health, 1-874004-64-4, £15.00

A comprehensive guide to getting community care services, the law and how to complain or take legal action if things go wrong.

Dementia: Money & Legal Matters: a guide for carers (booklet), Alzheimer Scotland—Action on Dementia, 0-948897-20-1, £1.50 (single copies free to carers)

Covers planning for the future, benefits, community care rights and financial assessments.

Facing Dementia: useful information for people with dementia (booklet), Health Education Board for Scotland, free from Health Promotion Departments and the Dementia Helpline

Information on practical arrangements and coping with feelings for people who have been told they have dementia.

Getting Help from your Doctor (booklet), Alzheimer Scotland - Action on Dementia, 0-948897-22-8, £1.00 (single copies free to carers)

Answers questions such as, 'Can I talk to the person's doctor about my worries?', 'How is dementia diagnosed?', 'How can a GP help the person with dementia and the carer?'

Getting Local Action on Dementia: a resource pack for campaigners, Alzheimer Scotland—Action on Dementia, 0-948897-19-8, £10.00

Help with ideas for action and information on how organisations work, for anyone who wants to campaign to improve policies and services for dementia.

Incontinence and inappropriate urinating by Graham Stokes, Winslow Press, 0-86388-056-8, £8.55

Practical guidance on coping with continence management.

Keeping Safe: a guide to safety when someone with dementia lives alone (booklet), Heath Education Board for Scotland, free from Health Promotion Departments and the Dementia Helpline

This book is also useful for carers of people with dementia who do not live alone. It looks at how to assess what is a risk, balancing risks and freedom and independence for people with dementia and practical steps you can take to help someone be safer.

Living in the Labyrinth: a personal journey through the maze of Alzheimer's by Diana Friel McGowin, Mainsail Press, 0-9518684-2-8, £12.95

The author of this brave and powerful book was diagnosed with early-onset Alzheimer's disease in 1991.

Looking at Alzheimer's: an introduction to the disease and how it affects peoples' lives (video), Alzheimer's Disease Society, £10.00

For new carers, relatives of people with dementia and anyone who would like to know more about the progress of the disease and the demands it puts on carers.

My Journey into Alzheimer's Disease: helpful insights for family and friends by Robert Davis, Tyndale House Publishers (US), 0-8423-4645-7, available from Dementia Services Development Centre £4.50

The author was a minister in Miami and wrote this book after his own diagnosis of Alzheimer's disease. It is the story of his personal spiritual journey through the disease.

Person to Person: a guide to the care of those with failing mental powers by Tom Kitwood and Kathleen Bredin, Gale Centre Publications, 1992, 1-870258-27-4, £6.00

Written for both carers and professionals, this book is a clearly written and person-centred approach to caring.

Screaming and Shouting by Graham Stokes, Winslow Press, 0-86388-043-6, £8.55

Practical guidance on coping when someone with dementia screams and shouts.

Sexuality and Dementia: Carers' Perspective (video), Dementia Services Development Centre, £9.00

A small group of carers discuss how dementia affects peoples' sexual lives.

Surviving Dementia (video), Church of Scotland Video, 121 George Street, Edinburgh EH2 4YH, £9.99

Explains how dementia affects people with dementia and their carers and looks at the sorts of help offered in the community.

Talking Dementia: a tape for carers (audio tape), Alzheimer Scotland—Action on Dementia, £2.95

Explains dementia itself and looks at how to deal with problems, how to get help with caring and how to look after yourself as a carer. Includes interviews with carers and professionals.

Thinking About Moving into a Care Home (leaflet), The Scottish Office, free from the Dementia Helpline or local social work department.

Explains how the social work department can assess someone to see what type of home is suitable, and financial arrangements.

Understanding Dementia, by Alan Jacques, Churchill Livingstone, 0-443-04392-2, £16.50

Written by a consultant old age psychiatrist, this book explains dementia clearly and simply. Suitable for both carers and professionals who want to know more about the different causes of dementia and ways of coping with the problems the illness brings.

Wandering by Graham Stokes, Winslow Press, 0-86388-042-8, £8.55
Practical guidance on coping with wandering.

ACKNOWLEDGEMENTS

Coping with Dementia was revised and updated by Kate Fearnley.

Many people made suggestions and comments including carers, community psychiatric nurses, doctors, social workers, occupational therapists, psychologists, staff of Alzheimer Scotland—Action on Dementia and the Dementia Services Development Centre and others. Thanks are especially due to the following: Carole Archibald, John Armstrong, Liz Baikie, Gill Boardman, Averil Harrison, Kevin Hurst, Dr. Alan Jacques, Jane McGowan, Dr. Jane McLennan, Betty McNicoll, Margo Mason, Karen Thom, Hugh Toner, Dot Weaks.

NOTES